WHY BUDDHA NEVER HAD ALZHEIMER'S

A Holistic Treatment Approach Through Meditation, Yoga, & the Arts

Shuvendu Sen, MD

Health Communications, Inc.
Deerfield Beach, Florida

www.hcibooks.com

**Library of Congress Cataloging-in-Publication Data
is available through the Library of Congress**

© 2017 Shuvendu Sen, MD

ISBN-13: 978-07573-1994-5 (Paperback)
ISBN-10: 07573-1994-7 (Paperback)
ISBN-13: 978-07573-1995-2 (ePub)
ISBN-10: 07573-1995-5 (ePub)

Publisher: Health Communications, Inc.
        3201 S.W. 15th Street
        Deerfield Beach, FL 33442–8190

Cover design and interior design and formatting by Lawna Patterson Oldfield

CONTENTS

ACKNOWLEDGMENTS

Before any conviction comes courage. The courage to dream, to dare, or to unfold. To Marilyn Allen, my literary agent, former Vice President of Harper Collins and presently the creator of the Allen O'Shea Literary Agency, I owe that courage. I owe my courage to her vision when all seemed blurry as well as to her unfailing persistence and faith in refusing to surrender.

My gratitude to the entire HCI team, my newly found home. Especially to Christine Belleris, David Tabatsky, Allison Janse, and Ian Briggs for their profound input and guidance, at once professional and personal. Thanks also to Lawna Patterson Oldfield, for her beautiful design of the cover and the interior of the book. And of course to John Paine, who edited my proposal package to HCI.

To the talent and tenacity of my editor, Gabriella Oldham, I will remain infinitely indebted. It was an absolute pleasure interacting with someone who deeply understood the vagaries of a struggling manuscript.

I am grateful to my many colleagues and mentors who have shared their time and resources with me, including Dr. Jon Denninger (Chief of Mind Body Institute, Harvard University), Dr. Benjamin Rolin Doolittle (Program Director, Internal Medicine-Pediatrics Residency Program, Yale University School of Medicine), Dr. Constante Gil (former Program Director, Raritan Bay Medical Center), Dr. Ronald Brenner, (Chief of Psychiatry, Catholic Health Services), Dr. Rajkumar Singh, librarian Zina Kolker, Shyamasree Bose Majumdar for her pictorial contributions, and many others I am guilty of not remembering but thankfully acknowledge.

And, of course, without the unconditional and unflinching support from Paramita, my wife, my two angels, Shraman and Shrimoyee, and other countless friends, this book would not have seen the light of the day.

INTRODUCTION

All experiences are preceded by mind,
having mind as their master,
created by the mind.

—Lord Buddha

When I first met Mrs. Lisa Wolfe, she was well into her eighties. As she rolled into my room in a wheelchair, followed by what seemed to be the entire Wolfe dynasty, extending from sons and daughters to great-grandchildren, I was instantly taken by her buoyant presence, in spite of her stiff countenance. Her fragile eyelashes framed razor-sharp eyes that virtually spoke on their own. Her skin was surprisingly wrinkle-free and flawless. She broke into a sweeping smile the moment she entered.

"Pleasure meeting you, Mrs. Wolfe." I said, surprised by my own animated spirit, considering that she was my last scheduled patient after a long arduous day in my clinic and at the hospital.

Instead of replying, she questioned back, obviously referring to her last name.

1

"When was the last time you so graciously welcomed a two-legged animal?" she said, laughing out loud.

It turned out this was more of a social visit. Mrs. Wolfe was in a rush to leave, as she had a baseball game to watch that evening. Apparently, her previous primary care facility had closed. Mrs. Wolfe wanted someone closer to her home who "wouldn't retire or die" before her "own end comes." She had no major complaints, save for a nagging fatigue she attributed to her growing years.

Considering her age, the physical examination was outstanding. Her heart and lungs were clear and her belly was benign. Realizing that fatigue could be a manifestation of one or more of many hidden mishaps, I ordered a preliminary work-up and let her go. She winked at me as she was being wheeled out.

"If you can get rid of the darn fatigue," she said, "I will rewrite my will."

Her blood reports came back reasonably steady and I had little reason to ask for a revisit within the next three months. Two months down the road, however, I got a call from Janice, Mrs. Wolfe's granddaughter.

"I want to relay to you a strange happening concerning Grandma." Janice's voice had an undertone of panic.

"If it's an emergency, Janice," I said, "you should call 911 and bring her to my hospital."

Sensing her urgency, I did not want to waste any time.

"Nothing physical. It's just that last night she forgot where the switch of her ceiling fan was, and instead she was using her walking stick to move the fan. I thought that was very peculiar and wanted to let you know."

"Did you notice any forgetfulness on her part?"

"Not really. But she has been forgetting familiar names and objects."

"Since when?"

"For quite some time."

"I wish you had told me that at her last visit."

I was disappointed, to say the least.

"Could you bring her back? I would like to perform some additional tests."

When Mrs. Wolfe returned to my office, I performed the Mini Mental Status examination, an initial assessment of cognition and mental status that can be brief or more extensive, depending on the setting and level of concern. Systematically going through the various cognitive spheres, including attention and concentration, memory, language, visual-spatial perception, calculations, executive functioning, mood, and thought content, the test reaches a maximum score of 30.

Mrs. Wolfe failed with a score of 15. Not convinced, I pursued the Montreal Cognitive Assessment (MoCA) that has emerged as a preferred brief assessment tool, owing to its superior sensitivity in detecting mild cognitive impairment, as well as executive and language dysfunction. She failed that, too, with a score of 22.

Eventually diagnosed with Alzheimer's disease, Mrs. Wolfe continued to deteriorate, despite her run with psychiatrists, neurologists, half a dozen imaging studies, and more blood work. She was prescribed both of the major drugs available in the market for the treatment of Alzheimer's—tacrine and memantine. Neither drug touched her dwindling mind. The tipping point came when she struggled to recall my name on one of her return visits.

"You have brown skin, Doctor," she said. "You must be an Indian."

That was all she could muster when I quizzed her. She was still smiling radiantly, refusing to surrender to a disease rampant in its ascent. Grounded with a relentless dementia and frequent mood disorders that fluctuated from deep depression to virile temper, Mrs.

Wolfe soon sank into a whirl of nameless emotions, becoming a functional ruin behind her seemingly intact structural framework.

I sometimes wonder whether we physicians have missed the boat. In the deluge of endless CAT scans, MRIs, and PET scans, have we stopped using the primordial organs with which we started our practice of medicine—our eyes and ears, with a finger on the pulse? In our rush for a diagnosis, do we circumvent the very beholders of the disease? Does our maddening desire to know the brain make us overlook the impossible width and depth of the human mind? In a tragic twist of fate, despite medicine's incredible advances, competent, conscientious, and yet compassionate doctors have become an endangered species.

Nowhere is the cry for answers more poignant than with Alzheimer's disease. A terrifying spectacle sinks mind after mind, unbridled and untouched by any type of resistance thrown at it. This disease springs from an organ that is the least understood and felt in our body, one that robs a person of emotion and identity, transforming all humane faculties into an expressionless stare.

In Alzheimer's disease, the medical world is facing its hardest hour. Of all the diseases that continue to harass humanity, Alzheimer's holds hostage the very fulcrum of human existence: its *mind*. Far more surreptitious than a stroke or tumor that grows, flares, or strikes with characteristic visibility and grandiosity, by turning the brain into a bloody battlefield Alzheimer's is that serpent in the grass that doesn't give a hint of its existence in the air. Its deceptive presence evokes virtually no resistance, as it spews its venom virtually unchallenged. When the serpent finally decides to announce itself, the human brain has already turned into jelly, helpless as it yields to the serpent's sinking teeth.

Scientists and physicians have tried to defy it the way they always have—with imaging studies, molecular genetics, and the pharmaceutical industry. But we also realize that unlike other disorders that harp on certain organic traits, Alzheimer's deals with memory, the finest and the flimsiest of our faculties. For an entity as integral, infinite, and invisible as memory, a drug or procedure is as futile and redundant as a group of ants trying to grapple with a giant pizza.

So while stress can be managed, mood can be elevated, growth can be arrested, blood can be stalled, and a clot can be busted, memory cannot be revived with a single magic bullet.

The chatty familiarity of care, love, and affection do little to dent the fact that when it comes to cut-and-dry disease prevention, today's practice of medicine is still scratching the surface. Unlike any other organ, the brain remains the only one that has little control of the boundless possibilities of its own existence. Moving from consciousness, awareness, cognition, and metacognition, to motivation, intention, insight, and free will, the brain and mind arc seamlessly back and forth, exchanging each other's position as cause and effect.

Like the classical Achilles tendon of modern medicine, Alzheimer's disease highlights the shortcomings and incredible challenges of a branch of science that, despite its bludgeoning advances, thrives on external discoveries while completely ignoring the treasures from its own internal resources. The understanding that this disease is much more than a rusty brain that has dwarfed due to disuse makes one cringe at the limitless possibilities that might be leading to this tragic state of inertia. The overwhelming fact remains that unless we have a deeper understanding of how the mortal mind works beyond the configuration of the brain's anatomical landmarks, we will find it hard to tame a beast that revels in random invasions. In other words, unless we comprehend how we remember and relate, we cannot comprehend how we forget.

Making matters more ominous are the rapidly emerging concepts that Alzheimer's is not just about loss of memory; nor does it involve only the sufferer. Almost like an infectious disease, it trespasses from the patient to the caregiver. A singular disease turns into a family affair that is at once vicious and aggressive. As a result, depression, agitation, personality changes, stress, and allied cognitive disorders become inevitable ingredients of a complete package for both the patient and those caring for the patient.

To put it succinctly, this is one fiend whose taming calls out for not just neuroscientists but masters of philosophy, sociology, physics, and I dare add, spirituality.

Let us move into facts and figures because numbers tend not to lie. Simple statistics will tell us that we are at the threshold of an epidemic. Current research from the National Institute on Aging estimates that between 2010 and 2050 the number of people age sixty-five and older will more than double to 88.5 million, or 20 percent of the population. In the United States alone, by 2025, the number of people age sixty-five and older with Alzheimer's disease is estimated to reach 7.1 million. By 2050, that number may reach 13.8 million. Between 2016 and 2025, every state and region across the country is expected to experience an increase of at least 14 percent in the number of people with Alzheimer's, due to increases in the population who are age sixty-five and older.

The financial numbers are even worse. Undoubtably, Alzheimer's is the most expensive disease in the world. Right now in the United States, we are spending nearly 160 billion dollars in Medicare and Medicaid for those with Alzheimer's. By 2050, we are looking at spending 1,092 trillion dollars if we do not put the brakes on this nightmarish disease.

As with other diseases, FDA-approved drugs specifically for the treatment of Alzheimer's, like donepezil, galantamine, and rivastigmine, rolled in with great expectations, carrying loads of promises while riding on various hypotheses tinkering with the brain's neurotransmitters. Each took their own turn being best sellers, yet none have been able to halt Alzheimer's in its relentless, destructive march.

It soon became inevitable to look beyond pharmaceutical drugs and seek other modes of management. Almost justifiably, the scientific world turned its attention toward holistic avenues. Meditations, yoga, music, and virtual reality have all emerged as serious considerations. Of these, mediation and yoga, in particular, steeped in centuries of experience, quickly took center stage. What began as spiritual practices from the deep recluses of mountains and forests soon promised firm pathways of human relief. As an inward journey, meditation took a completely different path to address various cognitive challenges.

The rich stillness and natural composure of Buddha (variously called Gautama or Siddhartha)[1] are not just a reflection of a spirit in awakening. It is more a state devoid of disturbances, both emotional and structural. Buddha lived well beyond the age of eighty and passed away, fully conscious, in untouched mindfulness. It is difficult to imagine Buddha in any pose other than his meditative self. One experiences an embryonic awakening at the sight of Buddha sitting for thousands of years, cross-legged, with an unbent and fluent spine, a pair of eyes closed in inward contemplation, a phlegmatic face beholding a body in wonderful stillness.

---

1 According to Mahayana tradition various Buddhas belong to various *kalpas* (Sanskrit word meaning aeons or a long period of time). The present Gautama belongs to the *bhadrakalpa* (Auspicious Aeon)

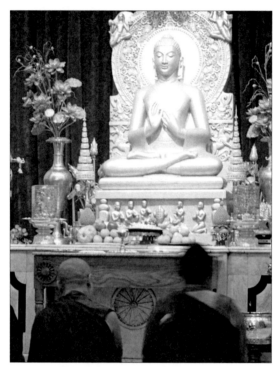

The classical meditative pose of Lord Buddha.

Yet, he is not the only one. A cursory look around, spanning across national boundaries, up mountain ranges, or deep into forest recluses, will reveal similar postures, soaked in demure composure and echoless silence. Their common bond is not just in the posture but in a continuity of life, unperturbed by the march of time. These men and women live long and yet die young as complete masters of their destiny and merit us revisiting their microcosm.

∽

William Camden, antiquarian, historian, and topographer, is credited for the birth of the English, saying, "All the proofe of a pudding is in the eating."

Modern medical management falls under this spell of evidence-based medicine, where nothing is considered standard unless it can be held in our palms and felt. In other words, any idea from an exalted imagination must go the route of hypothesis, using methods, materials, and statistical significance, as well as the four phases of trials under the scrupulous eyes of pharmaceutical industries, before being called therapeutic. No one doubts or should challenge the authenticity of today's practice of medicine because we are in the business of saving lives and there cannot be any room for opinions and procrastinations.

But we have a caveat here.

What if the methods and materials used as objective procedures are not advanced enough? Would they be able to capture the finest ideas with shimmering curative potential? Probably not. Therefore, to disregard an idea or a hypothesis as unscientific and not evidence-based could be either secondary to the shallowness of the idea or a reflection of a technology that has yet to sharpen its nails.

To me, a graver problem lies elsewhere. However lifesaving they may be, no drugs are exactly angels in the sky. First come side effects, some subtle and manageable. The more serious ones, called adverse effects, demand a second set of drugs to combat them. A roulette of more drugs follows. Then comes resistances and the peril of drugs randomly resistant to their effects and peculiar to every individual. Tolerance becomes another menace—and more so in the field of psychiatry.

For example, alprazolam is a particularly overused and abused drug, prescribed for treating anxiety. It is no longer the prerogative of the psychiatrist. Internists, family physicians, and even surgeons, prescribe it to their patients. Almost anyone can take this drug. In a dog-eat-dog society where anxiousness is so easily legitimized, alprazolam knocks at every door.

With its first appearance, a worry-free world whirled in ecstasy. Then came tolerance. A 0.5 milligram dose that removed the anxious edge became futile after six-months of daily use. A one milligram dose flourished for a while, until a second drug followed or an escalation in dosage of the same drug. A shortsighted, drug-dependent, scientific fraternity stopped thinking beyond the next product. A study of the countless drugs that floated into the pharmaceutical system, and the countless trials that utterly failed to validate their lengthy claims, would point to a method that is either utterly lopsided or lacking in vision.

Deeper philosophical thoughts pose as practical questions:
How can consciousness be scientifically reproduced?
Why are things beyond science not considered scientific?
How scientific are the scientific materials used for judgmental purposes?

If faculties as subjective and subtle as those belonging to the human mind are to be made evidence-based, then science might have to shrug off the dogmas and demons that threaten its own thought process.

The birth of holistic medicine was not just to complement the chronic fatigue and frailties of mainstream medicine. It was more a necessity in a health management system, where drugs, like momentary rebels, rise and fall, due to a defect or a deficiency.

Born in British-occupied eastern India, in what was then East Bengal, Grandma came from a well-to-do family. But the 1940s were troubled times. Revolt was brewing from all corners. Subhash Bose, a maverick who pledged armed resistance against the rulers, captured the imagination of the common mass and Grandma joined the fight, thundering the podium against the political atrocities of the British. She donated all her jewelry and wealth in the pursuit of freedom.

The retaliation was quick and decisive. Her husband, a renowned gynecologist, was stripped of his state job. In one stroke, a family of eight plunged into abject poverty. Very soon after, Grandfather died. A widow at the age of forty-two, with six half-fed children, Grandma decided to cross the border into West Bengal.

What she did next was remarkable and quite unthinkable for those times. While working and raising her children almost singlehandedly, Grandma turned to writing during her private times, devoting herself to writing stories, verses, and songs. Schools adopted her stories and publishers loved her free-flowing rhythmic verses. This was quite unbelievable during a time when men ruled the earth, while women were measured by the number of children they delivered and raised. Grandma's children became respected professionals in their various fields. She did not need to find a second companion. Books had become her retreat and refuge.

It came as a shock when she was found missing one evening. A panic-stricken family searched the streets of Calcutta. When she was eventually found close to midnight on a dead-end street, she was undressed, exposed by the moonlight. She seemed frozen, suspended in time and space, swaying back and forth for a few meters. When she was brought home, Grandma had slipped into a completely different persona. All her familiar faces seemed to have faded into oblivion. Looking in the mirror, she could not recognize herself. Over the next few weeks, she stopped basic functioning. The volumes of her verses and other writings gathered dust. Back then, there was little in terms of the standardized scores we use today. There was no Mini Mental score, no Montreal Cognitive Assessment scores. Alzheimer's was just making her presence felt.

I was one of Grandma's favorites. She was hell-bent on making me a poet. But Grandma spent her next ten years trapped in her own emotional confinement—powerless to live, yet powerless to die. When she died at the age of eighty-two, I had entered sixth grade. Years later, well into my medical journey, I wondered at the suddenness of it all. How could a brain of such superior intellect shut down so quickly? What triggered such an agonizing collapse? Did Grandma see it coming?

Thirty years down the road, we are still asking the same questions.

∞

If by default William Camden is the father of twentieth century medicine, then by birthright German scientist Hans Berger is the father of twenty-first century neuroscience. The founder of the electroencephalogram and the inventor of various brain waves, Dr. Berger opened the floodgate of a field of research that until then had drawn little attention beyond derision and ridicule. What started off as an electrocorticogram on a seventeen-year-old boy on July 6th, 1924, became a mind-bending gateway to enter the human brain.

Meditation before Hans Berger was at best a cult, an eastern ritual lacking science and sophistication. In the early days of the century, when the first faint trickle of the benefits of meditation reached the scientific society, there was nothing too cerebral to boast of in the world of technology other than a lumbar puncture, pneumoencephalography, and ventriculography to detect the "sick states" of a brain. CAT scans, sophisticated versions of an MRI, or Positron Emission Tomograms (PET), were still a far cry away at that time.

Sometime in the early 1950s, Das and Gastaut studied seven Indian yogis who performed a type of yoga called Kriya Yoga. Their observations on the electrical activities of these yogi brains would go down as the first in an endless series of fascinating results the medical fraternity would witness time and time again. Not surprisingly, the authors of the earliest articles held onto EEG as the only methods and materials to project their experimental results. In their landmark article "Variations in the Electrical Activity of the Brain,

Heart and Skeletal Muscles During Yogic Meditations and Trance," published in the prestigious peer-reviewed journal *Electroencephalography and Clinical Neurophysiology*, they successfully showed the high-frequency patterns of beta waves in yogis in deep meditation that was followed by the emergence of alpha waves toward the end of the meditative state.

A quick probe into the function of the beta waves would instantly draw our attention and interest. The voice of beta can be described as that nagging little inner critic who gets louder the higher one comes into range. The literature is clear on this. At a fundamental range, beta brain waves are associated with normal waking consciousness and a heightened state of alertness, logic, and critical reasoning. It only means that for a brain subjected to functional degeneration, anything that will enhance its beta waves should, and must be, life-saving. Even at this rudimentary level of research, we are tempted to adopt beta waves as a fierce ally of a brain struggling to retain its retentive power.

Alpha waves are more interesting, and in the context of meditation, priceless. Appropriately known as Berger waves, they indicate a state of mind that is phlegmatic, free of upheavals, and pristine. To those in love with meditation, this becomes their love child, born and beckoned at will.

The redoubtable eye of the storm has been the emerging concept of Mild Cognitive Impairment (MCI). It is a prelude to the ultimate tragic drama—a nascent, silent slide toward the inevitable. So slender and subtle, we let it pass through our fingers unaware, almost seeking comfort from its non-threatening sound.

Many loosely-related terms have been used to describe constructs similar to or perhaps even the same as MCI: incipient dementia, isolated memory impairment, dementia prodrome, minimal Alzheimer's disease (AD), predementia AD, prodromal AD, and early Alzheimer's disease. Like a spy on the run changing disguises in each new situation, the terminologies change, yet most of these definitions do not fully overlap with the definition of MCI.

In 2013, in a move to break away from the ever-thickening soup of circling terminologies, the construct of mild neurocognitive disorder was introduced in the *Diagnostic and Statistical Manual of Mental Disorders (DSM-5)* (5th ed.). Mild neurocognitive disorder is very similar to MCI as defined, and for the clinician, the two entities are equivalent. It refers to a condition involving cognitive impairment in one or more domains, often memory, with relative preservation of activities of daily living and the *absence of dementia.*

The absence of dementia makes this mild cognitive impairment phase such a powerful and tempting arena for a head-on duel. Neuropathological studies have suggested that MCI represents an early clinical expression of age-related neurodegenerative disease. Several autopsy studies have found that individuals with MCI have Alzheimer's disease pathology that is intermediate in severity—between normal controls and persons with a more advanced state. At a stage where the damaging neurofibrillary tangles of advanced Alzheimer's have not settled in, or the destructive proteins called *tau* have not completely taken over the brain, we have a perfect template to tame the tempest.

Considering this possibility, could we channel the boundless capabilities of meditation to confront and prevent Alzheimer's? Even before we attempt to answer, we need to revisit the infinite capabilities of the disease, itself.

⚭

The following examples highlight why the pathogenesis of Alzheimer's Dementia is not just about memory loss and mood disorders, but possibly a far more intricate and skewed event.

A Hungarian-born American film director and professor at New York University, Karl Bardosh is also a proud son of a courageous mother who fought the Nazis tooth and nail before her miraculous escape from a fatal capture. Shot in the back by a German bullet, she fell face down in the river and drifted, pretending to be dead until she floated to safety on the opposite shore. Years later, safe and sound in her adopted land in the United States, she succumbed to Alzheimer's and hid herself in the bathtub every time she heard the screaming sirens of New York police cars, thinking they were German bullets.

I once heard an equally poignant story from Jonathan Gray, an attorney, producer, and an adjunct faculty at New York's Columbia University, in his rustically decorated office in the Chelsea district of Manhattan. He switched on his cell phone to show me a video clipping of him attempting to converse with his mother, who crippled with Alzheimer's, was seemingly comfortable yet removed from reality with her typical nonchalant expressions. Out of the blue she looked to her left, where a mirror hung on the wall. On seeing her son's image, she shouted as if suddenly awakened, "Hi Jonathan." Before he could erupt in celebration at her unexpected recognition, she turned back to face her son and resumed her flat expression.

Why and how did Jonathan's mother recognize the image and not the real face? What was common in both the whistling bullets and the police sirens that drove Karl's mother to hide in the bathtub? Were these reactions coincidental, or did some unknown crevice of the mind suddenly tap into another level of awareness?

These events beg a different management approach, one that can traverse beyond the organic structure of a brain into the complex realms of a mind, where consciousness, subconsciousness, cognition, and metacognition, are taken into consideration in a process that will tread from the coarsest to the finest of our faculties. Unlike any other disease, Alzheimer's seems to affect the entire gamut of our cognition and can hardly be rectified by a hit-and-run drug.

As we struggle with the increasingly complex nature of this disease, it becomes imperative for us to reexamine the fundamentals and implications of the ancient practice of meditation. This is imperative because meditation, almost like some commercial product, has passed through the hands of spiritual leaders, scholars, philosophers, scientists, and even politicians, who have defined and used it at their discretion.

The term *meditation* now reflects a broad variety of practices— from techniques designed to promote relaxation to exercises with more far-reaching goals, such as a heightened sense of well-being. For a practice so flexible and open-minded, it is important to be specific about the type of meditation practice we are investigating. Scientifically, meditation can be conceptualized as a family of complex strategies developed for different purposes, including the cultivation of well-being and emotional balance. This helps us to crystallize specifically on Focused Attention (FA) meditation and Open Monitoring (OM) meditation.

Simplistically, FA meditation entails voluntarily focusing attention on a chosen object in a continued, persistent fashion. OM meditation involves non-reactively monitoring the content of experience from moment to moment, primarily as a means to recognize the nature of emotional and cognitive patterns.

In many instances, OM meditation initially can involve the use of FA training to calm the mind and reduce distractions, but as FA advances, the cultivation of the monitoring skill becomes the main focus of practice. The aim is to reach a state in which no explicit focus on a specific object is retained. Instead, one remains only in the monitoring state, attentive moment-by-moment to anything that occurs in the experience.

These two common styles of meditation seek the same depth as the quiet waters of the ocean, and both owe deeply to the traditions of Buddhist *Vipassanā* and *Mahāmudrā*—benedictions from the fig tree where Siddhartha once sat.

In order to consider meditation as "evidence-based medicine," we need concrete results. Personally, I have tried holistic treatment in my practice with heartwarming outcomes.

Michael Wallace, a retired schoolteacher, had been struggling with numbers, words, and basic executive skills, like counting and reasoning—a painful paradox for someone who prided himself on his mathematical faculty. He knew things were not right when, one afternoon, he had to strain hard to call a pen a pen—an object close to his heart, specifically a Sheaffer ballpoint pen he had received for winning an essay competition 30 years earlier. For a person of such intellect, this was ominous. However, he was still driving on his own and had no problems maneuvering the emotional complexities of a retired life. But once in a while, numbers eluded him, as did familiar objects and faces. He had been to his family physician. Some trademark blood tests were ordered, including Vitamin B_{12}, a thyroid panel, a Rapid Plasma Reagin test (RPR), a blood test notoriously over-ordered by physicians and hellishly biased with syphilis, and all came back normal.

Predictably, Michael was sent to a psychiatrist. More diagnostic tests followed but no firm diagnosis could be reached. According to the pundits, Michael fell somewhere between

"early onset Alzheimer's" and "Unspecified Dementia." No firm diagnosis meant no firm medications. As would be expected, true to the spirit of the "defensive medicine" practiced in today's world, a couple of anti-anxiety and multivitamin medications were prescribed.

Nothing happened or changed in Michael's lifestyle, save some periodic forgetfulness. Unaffected by the prescribed pharmacotherapies, Michael sought a mind-body expert. He was taught the virtues of meditation and yoga. These were new to him and he needed time to look them up by himself.

Michael came to me for a fourth opinion. I told him that when meditation is pursued in a simplistic way it does not have adverse effects, resistance, or tolerance, which are the three perils of modern medication. So why not try an age-old practice that has withstood the test of time?

Michael eventually approached a certified meditator and pursued it diligently. Within six months, he started showing improvement in his cognitive skills. Like Michael, many individuals across the globe have been benefitting immensely from meditation.

Are these success stories anecdotal, incidental, or isolated events with little relevance or credibility? Is meditation simply a placebo, or are there any causal associations?

It is here that we take refuge in the strength of occidental science, trying to cushion an oriental treasure that is striving to find its footing in the medical world. What was felt and sought is now pursued rigorously. From doctors obsessively pelting prescriptions to healers seeking new pastures beyond drugs, the recent pendulum swing across the arc of medical practice has been wonderful. Not very many years back, words and concepts like *consciousness* and *metacognition* were considered untouchables. If drugs could do the trick; if signs and symptoms plaguing the patient could be subdued, why bother stepping beyond? We basked for years under the glory and power of pharmaceutical industries. I, among millions of other physicians, prescribed, eyes shut, in complete faith to the pill that rolled out of a trial.

The sounding board came from Dr. John Denninger, MD, PhD, and Director of Research at the Benson-Henry Institute for Mind-Body Medicine at Massachusetts General Hospital. A strong advocate of meditation and yoga for wellness, he recently cited Dr. Herbert Benson from Harvard Medical School, who along with Drs. Robert Keith Wallace and Archie F. Wilson, researched individuals undergoing Transcendental Meditation (a form of chanting meditation). Titled "A Wakeful Hypometabolic Physiologic State" and originally published in the 1971 issue of *American Journal of Physiology*, this landmark research showed decreased oxygen consumption, increased carbon dioxide elimination, and higher respiratory rate, among other parameters—all indicators of a state of sustained calm uniformly found in those who practiced meditation.

These results propelled numerous scientific endeavors by the Mayo Clinic, Johns Hopkins, Harvard University, and a multitude of research institutions around the globe. By the turn of the twenty-first century, holistic approaches were formally signaling the advent of meditation as a powerful tool of patient care, both as a primary and complementary mode of treatment.

Let us entertain some examples.

In a well-designed, randomized trial conducted at Beth Israel Deaconess Medical Center and Harvard Medical School, patients with MCI showed positive effects after practicing Mindfulness Based Stress Reduction (MBSR), a standardized mindfulness meditation and yoga intervention. Results showed improved mindfulness skills, well-being, interpersonal skills, acceptance and awareness of MCI, decreased stress reactivity, and general group benefit. In fact, results from the Harvard Medical Center have been very encouraging when daily 15-minute guided mindfulness meditation sessions are "prescribed" to individuals affected with stress and depression.

Stress, as we will address in depth in subsequent chapters, is an inevitable key factor in the precipitous arrival of Alzheimer's and many other cognitive deficiencies. For compelling reasons, it has been the subject of intense research. In studies conducted by scientists at the University of California at Los Angeles (UCLA) under the leadership of Elizabeth Blackburn, the Australian-American Nobel laureate who currently heads the Salk Institute for Biological Studies, patients who practiced twelve minutes of daily yoga meditation for eight weeks showed significant improvement in stress-induced aging of the brain cells.

Another set of scientists from the Columbia College of Physicians pointed to similar effects of yoga and meditation in treating stress-related medical illnesses, anxiety, Post-Traumatic Stress Disorder (PTSD), depression, and substance abuse. Parallel studies conducted at the Landstuhl Regional Medical Center in Germany have shown equally beneficial results.

At Johns Hopkins University, *Kirtan Kriya* (a form of chanting yoga where a word or *mantra* is repeatedly uttered) has been used successfully in decreasing stress levels (shown as a reduction of inflammatory proteins) while increasing cerebral circulation. A meditation chanting program originating from Kundalini Yoga (a school of yoga that promotes awareness), *Kirtan Kriya* involves a twelve-minute daily chanting of specific mantras, along with specific finger poses (mudras).

Can these institute-based research trials be implemented as clinical therapies to prevent Alzheimer's?

"They certainly suggest benefits," says Dr. Denninger. "What is really needed is a 'longitudinal study' comparing minds with and without the practice of meditation. That would find gold."

Denninger's optimism begs us to turn our attention to Matthieu Ricard, a French genetic scientist turned Buddhist monk. Son of French philosopher Jean-François Revel and artist Yahne Le Toumelin, Matthieu was born in Paris, France in 1946 and grew up among its intellectual and artistic circles. Showing precocious intellect since boyhood, he earned a Ph.D. in cell genetics at the renowned Institut Pasteur, under the Nobel Laureate Francois Jacob.

When he was barely twenty years old and at the threshold of achieving so much, Matthieu, unexpectedly traveled across the continent to India to meet great spiritual masters from Tibet. This was not the only time people had traversed with effortless ease from deep-rooted science to deep-toned spirituality. Matthieu Ricard made that transition from the busy alleyways of Paris to the sublime ranges of the Himalayas, where he met up with and took refuge in the hearth of the Dalai Lama. Since 1989, he has been serving as the French interpreter for the Dalai Lama. He is an active member of the Mind and Life Institute, an organization dedicated to collaborative research between scientists and Buddhist scholars and meditators. He is engaged in research on the effect of mind training and meditation on the brain at various universities in the United States and Europe.

Around the same time, another scientist was embarking on a similar journey outside the realm of mainstream research. As the William James and Vilas Research Professor of Psychology and Psychiatry, and as University of Wisconsin's Founder of the Center for Investigating Healthy Minds at the Waisman Center, Richard J. Davidson was exploring the neural bases of emotion and emotional style and methods to promote human flourishing, including meditation and related contemplative practices. Named as one of the 100 most influential people in the world by *Time Magazine* in 2006, his studies have encompassed persons of all ages, from birth though old age, including individuals with emotional disorders, such as mood and anxiety disorders and autism, as well as expert meditation practitioners with tens of thousands of hours of experience. Taking full advantage of an era of rapidly advanced technology, Dr. Davidson has used a wide range of methods, including different varieties of MRI, positron emission tomography, electroencephalography, and modern genetic and epigenetic methods.

It was not at all surprising that Matthieu Ricard would fall under the radar of Richard Davidson. As a part of research on hundreds of advanced practitioners of meditation, Dr. Davidson wired up the monk's skull with 256 sensors at the University of Wisconsin.

The scan results were breathtaking. Ricard's brain when meditating on compassion produced a level of gamma waves—those linked to consciousness, attention, learning, and memory—"never reported before in the neuroscience literature," according to a euphoric Davidson.

The scans also showed excessive activity in his brain's left prefrontal cortex compared to its right counterpart, which researchers believed gave Matthieu an abnormally large capacity for happiness and a reduced propensity towards negativity. Research into the phenomenon, popularly known as "neuroplasticity," is still in its infancy and Ricard and other leading scientists have been at the forefront of ground-breaking experiments across the world.

"We have been looking for twelve years at the effect of short- and long-term mind-training through meditation on attention, compassion, and emotional balance," Matthieu said. "We've found remarkable results with long-term practitioners who did 50,000 rounds of meditation, but also with three weeks of twenty minutes a day, which of course is more applicable to our modern times."

Fortified with the latest and sassiest of modern technologies, including functional magnetic resonance imaging (fMRI), appropriate pulse sequences (to acquire data rapidly), fiber optic stimulus delivery devices (to present visual stimuli to subjects), and a high-density recording system using between 64 and 256 electrodes on the scalp surfaces, Matthieu went on to interrogate the neural correlates of FA meditation in experts and novices. Multiple brain regions were targeted for mapping activations on both meditators and novices.

The results were fascinating. Compared to novices, those who did extensive FA meditation training required minimal effort to sustain focus. They also found that advanced levels of concentration are associated with a significant decrease in emotionally reactive behaviors that are incompatible with stabile concentration, and that attention as a trainable skill could be enhanced through the mental practice of FA meditation.

Meanwhile, drug-shy scientists continued to push the boundary and happily ventured into the realms of music and virtual reality. Intriguing studies have emphasized the beneficial effects of Mozart's *Sonata for Two Pianos in D Major* on cognitive aspects of human brain (the so-called Mozart Effect). In research conducted by the Department of Neurology of Kaohsiung Medical University in Kaohsiung, Taiwan, dementia-screening indices, like the Mini Mental Status examination and Cognitive Abilities Screening Instrument (CASI), showed uncanny memory gains for Alzheimer's patients exposed to the Mozart Effect. As we will witness in subsequent chapters, music and even simple "touch" can become surprising friends to lost minds.

Promise has also come from emerging concepts of Virtual Reality (VR). Immersive virtual environments technology has been used in therapy for phobias, stress, anxiety, exercising, and memory problems. Research by the U.S. Army-Baylor University Graduate Program in Physical Therapy in San Antonio, Texas, found that persons with dementia who were placed in a virtual environment felt a sense of control as they enjoyed the interactions, and demonstrated little difficulty in maneuvering a joystick.

Needless to say, among all these invigorating concepts, meditation and yoga have captured the romantic mind. But what has lifted them to the level of serious consideration is the recognition of Alzheimer's major risk factors. In a field of science where nervous theories yield to others as a ritual, the understanding of stress, high blood pressure, high cholesterol, obesity, diabetes, and family history as strong risk factors for Alzheimer's remains a firm point of entry when it comes to grappling with the disease.

This is precisely where and why yoga and meditation emerge as helping hands—both observant and insightful. Modern times foster a lifestyle that spirals us out of our own existence. We seem to have lost the restrained elegance of a purposeful life. Nowhere are those hands needed more than now.

As I will highlight throughout this book, recent research has begun to show that meditation can rewire brain circuits to produce salutary effects, not just on the mind and brain but on the entire body, in a wondrous enhancement of brain connections involving axons, structures that connect various regions of the brain.

Unlike any other pharmaceutical drugs, the very fact that these techniques can endorse *neuroplasticity* on centers of focus and attention and increase alpha waves (responsible for enhanced cerebral attention and poise) make them superior options for treating a disease for which the world has little answer.

I asked Ron Brenner, Chief of Behavioral Health at Catholic Health Services of New York if he thought Mrs. Wolfe would have initially benefited from holistic approaches, like meditation.

"With no adverse effects," he said, "this could have been a viable option."

"And why?" Both the July sun and I were relentless in pursuit as we lunched and chatted one Sunday afternoon.

"Simply because meditation serves as a reserve or a resource that can be effortlessly used by the brain when challenged." Brenner's tone was instantly upbeat and authentic.

Dr. Benjamin R. Doolittle, Yale's Program Director of Combined Medicine and Pediatrics Residency Program, goes even further. He laments the fact that meditation, despite all that has been researched, is still an offering or option that is entertained only at the very late stage of a disorder.

Left to medications that were basically ineffective, Lisa Wolfe slipped into permanent and relentless Alzheimer's dementia. A firm alternative had existed all along, and if sensed early enough, a meditative approach might have turned the tide for her.

Suddenly, an audacious question beckons:

Can't we *propose* meditation as a preventive measure for Alzheimer's disease?

ALZHEIMER'S DISEASE: WHY WE ARE STILL SCRATCHING THE SURFACE

Gratitude is the memory of the heart.

—Jean Baptiste Massieu

Three ladies lived together, lodged in a plush suite of a senior center facility overlooking the ocean, and found a companionship more destined than designed. Mrs. Terry Behman spoke little, as her solemn expressions overrode her paucity of words. Margaret Mitchel spoke more, and her eyes darted like bullets. Lucy Adams served out of habit. Every dropped spoon was picked up without any fumble; every soiled finger was cleaned, and no spilled water escaped her attention. All three women had one thing in common: they all suffered from Alzheimer's. What prevailed was an unusual confluence of minds where all that mattered was embrace. Details became redundant.

If you review their histories, you would marvel at the present traces left behind. Terry is a retired high school teacher who ran the school with as much élan as she ran her house, with poise, grace, and determination. Margaret was one of America's earliest women pilots. Lucy served her entire life as a nurse. All three minds have now fallen behind. What remains are reflections of their wonderful choices: Terry's restrained expressions; Margaret's piercing eyes, and Lucy's unfailing gift of love and care.

These examples bring out the nature of Alzheimer's: unreliable and unsure. How much of the mind it bites away and how much it chooses to spare seem entirely left to the discretion of its whims. No matter how we try to formalize its ferocity with guidelines and templates, a new version inevitably emerges from right behind the curve.

In valiant yet vain efforts to taste the honey of success, scientists have been smashing one beehive after another, each of them clashing and colliding with the other, producing predictable outcomes from a disease in mindless turmoil.

Let me start with the Department of Psychology at Washington University in St. Louis, Missouri, to provide a better understanding of the endless perspectives scientists have adopted to trace this elusive predator.

Scientists there have examined personality changes in a longitudinal study using a Blessed Dementia scale. Of the 108 participants in the study, 68 received the clinical diagnosis of dementia after their entry into the study. The remaining 40 participants, who died during the study, did not have a clinical diagnosis of dementia. However, when autopsied, 14 of them received a neuropathological diagnosis of Alzheimer's. Based on the eight items of the Blessed Dementia scale, including increased rigidity, increased egocentricity, loss of concern or feelings for others, coarsening of affect, impaired emotional control and responsiveness, growing apathy, and purposeless hyperactivity, the participants' personality changes were measured. According to the results, 47 percent of the converters (those who became demented after joining the study) showed personality changes significantly before the clinical diagnosis of dementia—in sharp contrast to the nondemented group, who exhibited relatively preserved personalities. These changes included growing apathy, increased egocentricity, impaired emotional control, and increased rigidity.

A tempting question instantly emerged from these results: Can we use personality changes as a clinical marker of impending Alzheimer's? Should apathy or nonchalance be viewed as the first faint steps of a losing mind?

But if these are exciting and reasonable concepts, how do I rationalize Lucy's undisturbed care and affection, despite her advanced dementia? How do I overlook Margaret's intact personality expressed through her sharp eyes? Or Terry's restrained emotional quotient? Are they exceptions to the rule, or are we still scratching the surface?

We have opened a Pandora's Box. Numerous theories and hypotheses based on small longitudinal studies with little statistical significances are pouring in from all corners. Among all these impossibly moving targets, some facts remain—that Alzheimer's is an inexorable disease; that it can be varied in its presentation; that it can be slow and gradual or furious and relentless in pace and mood.

Dr. Bharati Sharma was one of those destined to be different and brilliant. An outstanding student in India, she boarded a plane to England at a time when in that part of the world, women in medicine were few and far between. As a member of the Royal College of Obstetrics and Gynecology, she worked with supreme credibility at Queen Charlotte Hospital and Kings Hospital in London before returning to her motherland to become a medical superintendent at a prestigious institute.

Despite her scholarly excellence, Dr. Sharma had little idea that her own mind would sink into Alzheimer's Dementia, grounding a mind that prided itself on taking care of mothers and infants in distress.

A single letter announced the arrival of Alzheimer's. In a letter to her husband, she started off normally, with "My dear husband," but as the letter progressed, quite suddenly and with no heralding sign, she lost her way and stumbled to a halt after a paragraph or two, ending as "Yours affectionately, Mother." A disease in a frenzied pace reversed her own identity in a matter of a few lines. There was no turning back. A doctor turned into a patient who would be need to be taken care of for the next twenty years. All was lost, except tragic remembrances, like when she scrubbed her hands, surgeon style, every time she sat for dinner. Painful reminders that she was once an outstanding doctor.

As of now, we have a grasp of the wide range of clinical manifestations that this disease can present but we have no sense of its timing. This could just be the nature of the beast—protean and whimsical. Future trials and studies would surely throw more light on this conundrum. Apart from memory loss that forms the fulcrum of the disease, impairment of executive functioning is a common presentation. However, this is not set in stone. The shortcomings may range from subtle to prominent, ranging from being less organized to being less motivated, and an individual may exhibit either state in varying magnitude. Yet as the disease progresses, the ability to perform complex tasks becomes seriously challenged.

Other signs and symptoms pour in randomly, almost in callous vengeance.

Dyspraxia, the art of performing learned motor tasks, sets in much later in the disease, long after memory and language have been hit. Can you button your shirt? How do you use a comb? Switch on the fan for me. Can you scoop jelly out of the bottle with a spoon?

Open-ended questions or instructions reflect an ability to perform multistep motor activities. But immersed in Alzheimer's, these abilities often falter, leading to dependency, frustration, pain, and compounding emotional agony.

By contrast, sleep disturbances can come early in the disease process, long before the mind has been dented. Fragmented sleep patterns, a quick-in/quick-out pattern of sleep, ending in prolonged periods of solitary nocturnal awakening with inevitable daytime drowsiness. Again, we must resist the temptation to take this early feature as a sign of impending Alzheimer's, for nearly anything disorderly in life can break the natural rhythm of sleep, including the normal, gracious aging of the mind and body.

Seizures, quite like sleep disorders, have a variable foothold in Alzheimer's. They occur in nine to 16 percent of patients and frequently involve the later stages of the disease.

A far more intriguing but unsubstantiated feature of the disease involves the olfactory function—our ability to smell the good, the bad, and the ugly. In a recent article published in *Neuropsychiatric Disease Treatment* (April, 2016), authors Yong-ming Zou et al. from the Department of Neurology at Tianjin Huanhu Hospital, Tianjin, People's Republic of China, delved deeply into the intricacies and sensitivities of olfactory dysfunction in Alzheimer's. Research and review of almost all scientific studies pointed out that an inability or reduced or distorted ability to smell can occur in the nascent stage of the disease.

Since as early as 1974, forty years of intense research have attempted to use olfactory dysfunction as one of the earliest clinical markers of this disease. The sensitivity of this disorder has been phenomenal, reaching about 100 percent in Alzheimer's. Yet, as with many of these biomarkers, specificity has been weak. In other words, even in a general healthy population, disturbed smell ability has been observed. In a major population-based cross-sectional study published in the *Journal of the American Medical Association* (*JAMA*), researchers from the School of Medicine at San Diego State University and the University of California have shown that the prevalence of olfactory dysfunction increases with aging. Statistically, patients who range from eighty to ninety-seven years of age had a 62.5 percent prevalence of olfactory dysfunction.

But the area in which Alzheimer's poses an especially considerable challenge is the "insight" faculty. Reduced insight is a common yet variable feature of this disease. An underestimation of one's own deficits with counter-explanations and alibis, almost as if to preserve one's self-dignity, becomes the most poignant feature of the suffering. Justifiably, the deficits are almost always observed by whomever the sufferer leans on most, which is very often a family member. But again, much like executive functioning, loss of insight is not a guaranteed presentation, and the consequences of these varied features go well beyond the primary disease. Those who manage to hold on to their insight sink into depression. By contrast, once the insight faculty is hurt, behavioral disturbances invariably take center stage in the form of agitation, aggression, wandering, and the psychotic effects of hallucinations, delusions, and—in severe situations—misidentification syndromes.

What increases the complexity is the observation that the simple physiological aging process can uncover all these behavioral disturbances. Dr. Rajkumar Singh, our institute's psychiatrist, who also carries an extensive research background, brought to my attention a study he had co-authored and presented at the 143rd annual meeting of the American Psychiatric Association in New York some years ago.

In that study, forty-five normal, healthy, young volunteers, between the ages of nineteen and thirty-five, were compared to forty-five normal, healthy, elderly individuals, ages sixty to seventy-eight. Both were administered a verbal list-learning task and self-rated scales of affective states to examine the relationship between emotional states and performance on a memory task. What Dr. Singh and his colleagues found was that the elderly group demonstrated strong correlations between poor verbal recall measures and heightened negative emotional states. In the elderly group compared to their younger counterparts, higher levels of negative emotional states were positively associated with poorer memory.

From a raw emotional point of view, misidentification carries the worst prognosis for the complete breakdown of relationships. The ripple effect eventually touches all—from the sufferer to the caregiver to the whole family.

I had always known Laura as one of the most devoted caregivers I had come across in my twenty-five years of patient care. John, her husband, was in my nursing home with a documented diagnosis of Alzheimer's, along with numerous other co-morbidities, ranging from coronary artery disease to high blood pressure to rampant diabetes that gave him severe peripheral vascular disease, eventually leading to a bilateral, below-the-knee amputation. But he was a sweetheart. Loss of memory, loss of legs—nothing could deter his joviality. He denied and defied all laws of Alzheimer's to show minimal behavioral and psychological symptoms—all except one, as I would discover much later.

After several sessions with both husband and wife, I gradually noticed strange but undeniable discrepancies in the couple's past lives. John vowed that Laura always loved Vivaldi and Chopin. When I approached her separately, Laura had no clue about either of those composers. John lauded Laura's outfits in her heyday, which were always blue, including the rim of the pince-nez she wore. Laura vaguely recollected those details. John named all the countries they had visited, yet Laura had a grounding fear of flights and heights.

I expressed my concerns to Laura, gently addressing issues pertaining to both health and law, for example, how difficult it would be to conduct behavioral and biofeedback sessions if facts did not gel, or how I might need to involve Human Resources if I was not convinced of their relationship. Our meeting was far from an interrogation, but I was persistent. Finally, Laura broke. The story she told was heartbreaking, to say the least, yet reflected how far Alzheimer's can go to derail and damage personalities.

Laura was not Laura, after all. She was John's second wife, Martha. John's first wife, the real Laura, had died of an unexpected cardiac arrhythmia. In the ensuing years, Martha had taken excellent care of a very crestfallen John, and they married and lived on happily—until slowly but surely Alzheimer's took over John's mind.

While memory loss was evident, misidentification became the leading feature. With his distant memory intact, John started seeing Martha as Laura. In extreme situations, he questioned Martha's demeanor and appearance because they did not fit into his construct of the departed Laura. Martha tried her best to battle the trauma until she could no longer sustain it, leading to an extreme, perverse transition when Martha *became* Laura. This was a new love story—intense, suffering, and deeply agonizing. It required intense counseling to convince Martha that by pretending to be Laura she was not only deepening John's dementia, she was also burning herself out.

This brings us to one of the fiercest challenges of Alzheimer's disease: caregiver burnout.

Haidi Behman, one of the brightest neurologists in our facility, had always prided herself on her subspecialty of epilepsy, which had become her passion, both for treating and teaching. About ten years ago, she suddenly encountered a bitter crossroads when she found her mother, Terry, in the kitchen completely clueless about the difference between a crockpot and a rice pot, two utensils she had been using for years. Haidi instantly recognized that something was terribly wrong. A predictable course followed: a quick Mini Mental exam followed by Namenda, a highly touted, brain-saving drug. Nothing happened. Terry did not improve or deteriorate; she simply plateaued. When her husband died, Terry turned completely silent and this may have been symptomatic of depression or worsening dementia.

This entire process changed Haidi from a neurologist to a caregiver, from someone who understood the disease to someone who felt its pain. The journey was rough for mother and daughter, and the stakes in their relationship became higher as the contrasts became starker. The woman who had virtually governed a neurologist now needed to be fed, seated in a reclining chair, and have her diapers changed.

This is Alzheimer's most powerful blow—turning a family into a portrait of sorrow and suffering. It almost justifies the absurdity of dementia and depression being considered as "infectious diseases."

A major landmark study by the Department of Psychiatry and Epidemiology at the University of Pittsburgh squarely addressed this threatening issue. Cross-sectional and longitudinal analyses were carried out involving 1,222 dementia patients and their caregivers to assess dementia patient suffering, caregiver depression, and the use of antidepressant medications. Called the REACH study (Resources for Enhancing Alzheimer's Caregiver Health), this multisite trial sought out various psychosocial interventions to measure their feasibility and the emotional impact on family caregivers living with and caring for patients of dementia.

The results were staggering. But even before we address the overwhelming statistics, we should be asking some fundamental and valid questions:

How do we measure suffering?

Is suffering relative?

Is it a completely personal issue?

How many times have we seen individuals flip out at the drop of a hat, while others remain stoic and nonchalant despite insurmountable hurdles? Or, even more astonishingly, they remain happy and resplendent in their expressions, despite facing incredible odds?

Researchers have argued that measurable universal manifestations of suffering exist, despite personal differences. Physical symptoms, like chronic or acute pain, nausea, and difficulty in breathing; psychological affects, like depression and anxiety; and from a holistic point of view, measures of internal harmony, meaning, and purpose of life, are all tangible and measurable factors.

In this study, suffering was assessed on the depression subscale of the Revised Memory and Behavior Problems Checklist (RMBPC). For example, caregivers were asked, "Within the past week has the patient . . . appeared sad or depressed, expressed feelings of hopelessness or sadness about the future, made comments about feeling worthless or being a failure?" and so on.

Baseline characteristics of both the Caregivers and Care Recipients were established based on nine items of the RMBPC, of which three assessed emotional distress (anxiety, sadness, and crying) and six assessed existential distress (worthlessness, failure, hopelessness, loneliness, talk of death, and self-threatening).

The researchers wanted to measure not only the demonstration of patient or caregiver emotional distress, but also the establishment of a direct relationship between patient suffering and caregiver well-being. Their findings were decisive and disturbing. Consistent with cross-sectional analysis, changes in perceived patient suffering had an independent yet inescapable bearing on caregivers, causing depression, anxiety, and immense emotional distress. Even worse, the more time they spent with the patient, the more their depression increased. It was not difficult to surmise that those who felt helpless in the face of their loved one's relentlessly progressive suffering demonstrated the deepest distress and depression, along with cyclical, sinking feelings of guilt, helplessness, and emotional trauma.

These finding provoke inevitable questions: Do we have enough understanding and knowledge of the reciprocal relationship between patient and caregiver? How do we break the cycle of suffering between patient and family caregivers? What branch of subspecialty is best suited to address this unique "infectious disease" where the "bug" is infinitely more subtle and vicious than any bacteria or virus?

In other words, who takes care of the caregiver?

One of the greatest casualties in modern medicine has been time. Caught in the cobweb of technological dependence, administrative influences, and legal threats, today's practice of medicine has increased the amount of time and energy doctors and staff must expend on thwarting external factors—to a point so overwhelming and exhausting that little time is left to spend in a patient's room—in those intensely personal interactions behind drawn screens. These are vulnerable moments for any individual, draped in a grim blue gown, barely tied at the back, when he or she is forced to lie on a cot where hundreds have been before, in a small, cheerless room with only a solitary window.

My hospital, Raritan Bay Medical Center, unfailingly provides a "Pride in Caring" comment card to demonstrate its commitment to those it cares for. It is not surprising that less than one percent of the Thank You cards from admitted patients involve any physicians. Unit assistants are mentioned, nurses are lauded, social workers are commended, yet an alarmingly low number of physicians are thanked, in spite of the fact that they have diagnosed pathologies, put in order requests, and dictated discharge instructions.

"Where are we going wrong?" I asked William Distanislao, Vice-President of Operations at our institute.

"Patients just cannot recall any personal moments with the doctors," he said.

A careful look at the *Improving the Patient Experience* daily email that Mr. Distanislao diligently runs every morning sheds a revealing light on a disturbing state of affairs. The impeccably designed layout has the following headings:

+ Standard registration
+ Helpfulness of registration person
+ Ease of registration process
+ Waiting time in registration
+ Standard facility
+ Comfort of waiting area
+ Ease of finding your way around
+ Cleanliness of facility
+ Standard test or treatment
+ Friendliness of staff
+ Explanations given by staff
+ Skill of techs/therapists/nurses
+ Staff concern for comfort
+ Staff's concern questions and worries
+ Standard personal issues
+ Our concern for privacy
+ Our sensitivity to your needs
+ Response/complaints during visit
+ Standard overall assessment

+ Staff worked together provide care
+ Overall rating of care
+ Likelihood of recommending

None of those items feature subheadings, such as:

Doctor's sensitivity to patient's needs
Doctor's concern for comfort
Explanations given by *Doctors*

These are strange but inevitable omissions, given the abysmal patient-doctor relationship of modern times.

The Accreditation Council for Graduate Medical Education (ACGME), a private nonprofit group that evaluates and accredits more than 9,000 residency programs across 135 specialties and sub-specialties in the United States, has established educational standards and common program requirements for all training programs. Their website states that in 2002, the ACGME launched a competency initiative called the Outcome Project. As a result of this project, ACGME identified six ACGME Core Competencies to be used by GME programs to evaluate their residents in training. The six ACGME Core Competencies are: patient care; medical knowledge; practice-based learning and improvement; interpersonal and communication skills; professionalism; and systems-based practice.

Something essential is obviously missing:

Why aren't senior folks accounted for in the six competencies?

The American Board of Internal Medicine (ABIM) runs the recertification program, whereby every medical graduate is required to take the Board certification exam every ten years. That accounts for medical knowledge, but what process do we have to re-measure the other five competencies, especially professionalism and communication skills? Do we have any mandated workshops, any simulated interactive programs? The answer is a resounding no, and this is exactly where we doctors falter in our patient care.

Consider the case of Richard Benedict, who suffered from severe back pain in the thoracic-lumbar region. While a preliminary X-ray did not reveal much, a subsequent MRI showed a severe spinal stenosis. I discussed various treatment options concerning conservative management and surgical intervention, and referred him to a neurosurgeon for a second opinion. Richard returned to my office, looking grim.

"What's the matter, Richard?"

"You didn't do a good job in your referral."

"Why? Didn't you like the neurosurgeon?"

"Nope."

I didn't respond immediately. I had a printout of the neurosurgeon's note, which was quite detailed. The physical examination, the assessment, and the plan were exquisite.

"I am reading his notes and he was pretty thorough," I said.

"You got it, Doc," said Richard. "That's what he did. He typed and typed. Hardly got up from the chair."

Electronic Medical Records (EMR), Computerized Physician Order Entry (CPOE), and Prescription Drug Monitoring Program (PDMP) are powerful terms that have replaced pen and paper. The cardinal motif is to eradicate errors caused by illegible handwriting and transcription of medical orders. Brilliant advances, no doubt. But the flipside means that words of warmth and assurances have yielded to monochromatic dictations over the phone. The consequences are fatal and far-reaching. Erosions occur from both ends—the science of medicine and the art of patient care.

Here is a personal example to drive home the point.

When Jennifer Walker was ushered into my clinic by her daughter, my undivided attention was on her. There were no surprises in her visit. Pam, my triage nurse, had already briefed me. The Walkers were new to our town and Jennifer needed a new doctor. She had a long-standing history of Alzheimer's, for which she was on Donepezil. She also had hypertension and diabetes, both under control.

Jennifer's hair was neatly tied into a ponytail. She wore a brightly colored gown with sparkling white shoes. She verbalized little. Most of her medical and non-medical background came from her daughter, who spoke rather slowly, almost tediously, with each word lingering before yielding to the next. There was nothing outstanding in Jennifer's physical examination. She smiled once in a while, more out of habit than any reflection of happiness. Predictably, she failed the Mini Mental exam. Jennifer's daughter reported that she initially thought her mother had marginal improvement in her cognition when on Donepezil, but now thought she was back to square one. Lack of initiation, will power, and energy was wrapped in an overall inability to recognize, recollect, or recall. Jennifer was 83, and had been in this state for the last ten years. I renewed her medications and let her go with some basic blood tests. I felt suffocated in my utter inability to make any difference to her present state of being. I knew that any prescribed assurances would provide little productive support.

Five days down the road, Pam stopped me in the corridor as I was entering the clinic.

"You remember Jennifer Walker, the elderly woman with Alzheimer's?" she said.

"Yes, why?"

"You remember her daughter?"

"Yes, vaguely."

"Did you know she gets treated for major depression?"

"No, How would I?"

I stopped right there as it all came back to me. Unlike Jennifer's prim and proper attire, her daughter had appeared disheveled and unkempt. In contrast to Jennifer's engaging silence, her words kept coming out strained and forced. Perhaps because of her compulsive wish to attend to her mother's state of suffering, she had slipped into her own relentless depression. In my own objective attention towards Jennifer's hapless state of living, I had completely missed out on the caregiver's plight. I didn't even recall her name.

You did nothing wrong.

You were professional.

You took care of your patient.

Those were my colleagues' responses when I addressed this issue with them. I knew they were all correct and meant well. I also realized where I had gone wrong. Call it dry objectivity, tunnel vision, or plain inertia to reach out, but the truth is, the mindset of today's medical practitioner has changed 90 degrees. From primary care to subspecialties, from being a family physician to a rushed internist, the practice of medicine has become narrower, steeper, and more irrevocably isolated.

Author Bruce Lee from Johns Hopkins University's Bloomberg School of Public Health emphasized the paramount importance of an internist in his article, "The Role of Internists During Epidemics, Outbreaks, and Bioterrorist Attacks." He argued that internists, with their broad range of medical knowledge, experience, and skills, are uniquely qualified to diagnose and treat a variety of potential health problems.

Potential. This is exactly where modern medicine has fallen flat. Billions of dollars have been spent on Alzheimer's disease for diagnosis, investigations, and infinite treatment options. But so far, any knowledge of its potential state *before* the disease forms is abysmally poor. The pipeline right now is completely dry. In other words, the first slender steps of the disease, its hushed and unseen hints, like a lull before the storm, have all been completely ignored.

These usurp guilty questions we cannot avoid: Can Alzheimer's be smelled before it becomes evident? Can we nip in the bud the ugly thorns that twist across the brain? Do we have a potential state where Alzheimer's growth can be halted before it gains strength?

In an age of slogans, catch-phrases and memes, no word or phrase has evoked more attention, seduction, and addiction than Mild Cognitive Impairment (MCI). In the ever-deepening mystery of an ever-emerging disease, we hold dearly onto this term. As of now, this is our only ray of hope, however unpredictable, controversial, and provocative. MCI has been declared completely heterogeneous in terms of clinical presentations, etiology, prognosis, and prevalence. It hangs somewhere in between the cognitive changes of aging and dementia—a fairly broad transit that warrants considerable judgment in making the cut between impairments that are physiological for the aging and reflective of an impending dementia.

The challenge does not end here. The basic concept of clinical impairment in daily living is an entirely individual notion. Such personal distinctions demand the finest clinical expertise, which cannot—and should not—rely solely on psychometric testing. This throws the challenge squarely at internists, family physicians, and physician assistants—the front-liners who invariably inherit these early moments of a disease. To the potential Alzheimer's patient, this becomes supremely challenging because, in many cases, they are left scuttling between a series of psychiatrists, geriatricians, and neurologists.

Despite all this chaos, we have been able to establish some basic facts of MCI. At present, we have zeroed in on two cardinal divisions: amnestic and non-amnestic.

As a precursor to Alzheimer's disease, amnestic MCI is the most common subtype, with a ratio of 2:1 compared to the non-amnestic variety. As you may have guessed, the amnestic variety was further broken down into Single domain and Multiple Domain types. It is relevant here to single out these individual constituents to better grasp what is existential and what is impending.

By definition, amnestic MCI (aMCI) refers to individuals with significantly impaired memory who do not meet the criteria for dementia. The breakdown was comprised of something like this:

Memory complaint (loss of familiar words, identities, and entities), not coarse and often subtle, in fact so subtle that the individual concerned does not even realize it. In most circumstances, they get corroborated by an informant.

Objective memory impairment (for age and education).

Preserved general cognitive function (behavioral and executive functions intact).

Intact activities of daily living (an individual can still drive, feed, and bathe at will).

Not demented (this is the best possible news!).

In contrast to Single domains, Multiple domains are only slightly impaired. Having said that, these individuals do sometimes encroach on the domain of cognitive functions and activities of daily living, making them more susceptible to converting into full-blown Alzheimer's.

What makes this information conflicting and difficult to manage is the corollary literature that actually reveals that a significant number of these individuals actually do not progress to Alzheimer's at all. Instead, they return over time to a baseline functional level.

Objectively, this is good news. Subjectively, this is a massacre because it means we do not have a firm grip on following the progress of Alzheimer's. We can understand the various paces of MCI to reach the final stage of Alzheimer's. But to have a subset of MCI that will not become Alzheimer's at any point of time thwarts all meaningful attempts to use it as a definitive starting point for any comparative studies.

In simple terms, to have any longitudinal studies, a uniform platform is necessary. Let us assume that we run a trial to compare meditation and one FDA-approved drug. Patients with proven MCIs would be the best candidates to begin the trial. End points could be set as (A) Patients who have converted to full-blown Alzheimer's, (B) Patients who are still within the range of continued MCI, or (C) Patients who do not even show any features of MCI.

The challenge comes at the very onset. If the trial includes a set of individuals who physiologically do not progress from MCI to Alzheimer's and we cannot identify who they are by any diagnostic means, we have no way to learn which individuals actually responded to either treatment. In other words, we cannot offer any superiority of one treatment over the other with any measurable statistical significance because we will also have a group consisting of non-converters to Alzheimer's. This is a huge stumbling block for any meaningful research, and a clear and firm indication of how difficult it will be to overcome this disease—unlike any other.

Fortunately, unless otherwise proved, those subsets of non-converters are few in number. so for the time being we can tread on the same path and persevere.

Variations do not end here. Along with the amnestic variety, a non-amnestic type is another possibility, where the primary feature is not memory loss but word-finding problems and prominently impaired reasoning, judgment, and/or problem solving.

For the sake of sanity, we can take the hand of the National Institute of Ageing and the Alzheimer's Association (NIA-AA) to chart out some method in this maddening discourse. According to these primary schools of thought, probable Alzheimer's Dementia is a syndrome that can be defined by the following characteristics:

✦ Slow gradual onset.

✦ Progressive worsening.

✦ A decline from a previous level of functioning and performing.

✦ Interference with ability to function at work or in usual activities.

✦ Cognitive impairment involving acquiring and remembering new information, reasoning and handling of complex tasks, visual spatial and language, and personality and behavior changes.

✦ Predominant amnestic presentation (impairment in learning and recall of recently learned information).

✦ Predominant non-amnestic presentations, including language presentations with word-finding deficits, visual-cognitive deficits, and dysexecutive presentations, as stated before.

What could be an *atypical* Alzheimer's disease?

Anything and everything. All possible permutations and combinations are possible here. It could have a sudden onset and be relentless, or it may not even progress an inch. Worse, it can be a mix of multiple other causes of dementia, including cerebrovascular, Lewy body type dementia (a slightly different type of dementia that also encompasses hallucinations or delusions and is named after Frederick H. Lewy, M.D., the neurologist who discovered it while working in Dr. Alois Alzheimer's laboratory during the early 1900s), Parkinson's related dementia, and any co-morbidities affecting the cognitive domain.

Mario Pedro is a classic example of how cognitive deficiencies can tease and torture us to no end. He was a sixty-eight-year-old homeless man who was picked up from the streets of Perth Amboy, New Jersey, and came in with a working diagnosis of altered mental status. His hair was disheveled, his face worn out, and his clothes smelled of dirt—all traits of someone who has been on the street for quite some time. He smelled of alcohol and had tremors. From his garbled speech, it was apparent he was of Latino lineage, and somehow, he uttered his name.

We pounced on the obvious diagnosis: altered mental status secondary to alcohol abuse. He was promptly put on Detox Protocol, the usual treatment to prevent reactions from alcohol withdrawal, consisting of folic acid, Librium, and thiamine. Interestingly, his alcohol level in the blood was not too high at 10 milligrams per liter.

Two days later, his tremors were gone and his speech was more lucid. Efficient nursing had cleared him of all the dirt he had brought to the hospital. I realized Pedro was a good-looking man, whose tired face broke into a wonderful smile every once in a while. His eyes were deep and searching. His body, now beaten, must have once been made of steel.

On the third morning, Pedro was put on a liquid diet and advanced to a soft diet the following day. He was soon out of bed to chair and seen walking down the corridor under the supervision of a physiotherapist. He was mildly ataxic and had to be held because he tended to sway a bit while walking. In an ideal situation, Pedro should have been discharged, either home or to a sub-acute rehabilitation facility. But he wasn't. We couldn't, because despite being successfully detoxified from alcohol abuse, Pedro continued to be thoroughly confused. He had an inclination to repeat words that he heard.

"Are you doing all right, Pedro?"

"Doing all right."

His tone carried no emotion.

"Anything bothering you?"

"Nothing bothering me."

Besides that, there was very little meaningful conversation. Pedro did not remember his family, his place of birth, where he'd lived, or his job—if he ever had one. I instructed my resident to take a Mini

Mental Score and Pedro came up with a dismal 15. There was no neurological deficit, in terms of involuntary movements, weakness of the limbs, or any cranial nerve deficits.

No one wanted to inherit this patient—someone whose past is unknown, whose future is uncertain, and whose present is confused. If the situation did not guide the providers, it certainly did not help the administrators, who predictably panicked. For case managers, social workers, and nursing supervisors—for essentially anyone linked to our hospital staff—Pedro became a problem no one wanted to solve. In situations like these, no one can point any fingers, as the hospital drains money like blood, social workers turn hoarse calling up nursing homes for any sort of disposition, while nurses simply do not know what care to mete out. Pedro ate, walked, sat, smiled, and slept in perfect precision—except he did not know anything else. A distraught hospital took to the media and placed an ad in the local newspaper.

The challenge lay beyond the social issues. Because we had no clue to his background, very little could be attempted in terms of any investigation or diagnostic approach. A CAT scan of the brain showed small dot-like lesions, indicating a likely microvascular disease. There were no other major issues, like tumors, pus, or blood.

Neurologists and psychiatrists joined the fray. While the former called it alcohol-related dementia, the latter held onto the MMSE score of 15 and called it "unspecified dementia." Yet donepezil, a major player in the treatment of Alzheimer's Dementia, was prescribed. As would be expected, a plethora of blood tests was showered on Pedro, none of which threw any light. And none of the drugs, including Donepezil, made any difference in his medical outcome.

Pedro had taken us back to pre-medieval times when, devoid of effective diagnostic tools, diagnosis became a figment of the imagination. I proposed an MRI of the brain, which is a more decisive test than CAT scan when it comes to detecting abnormalities at a deeper level of the brain. It was instantly turned down as redundant and not medically worthwhile because it would not change the course of events. A deeper cause lay behind the refusal, and a valid one. With no past medical or surgical history possible to be elicited from Pedro, we did not know whether he harbored any foreign body inside. This was essential to know, as a MRI cannot be done in the presence of any foreign material.

That's when I turned to Dr. Anthony Mark Musarra, our physician advisor. He possessed a keen intellect when it came to both diagnosis and disposition, and nursed that rare ability to step outside the box when making a firm decision. We talked about the ethical necessity of reaching a diagnosis for someone like Pedro whose pathology remained undetermined.

Only Anthony could have softened the rigid reluctance of the administration. He ordered the body screening required to detect the foreign body and all the imaging came out clean. Anthony joked about checking out a penile prosthesis to be absolutely safe. We did a MRI of the brain and within a few hours we received the results. The one phrase that stood out among the various possibilities was: cerebral amyloid angiopathy, recognized as one of the morphologic hallmarks of Alzheimer's disease. A definitive diagnosis was beyond any means as it lay on tissue studies typically obtained post mortem.

One of the serious and often fatal complications of this disease is intracerebral hemorrhage. It tends to be recurrent and frequently carries a poor prognosis. High blood pressure as a risk factor calls for thorough attention. Pedro's blood pressure ran on the higher side and complete control was started soon after, with multiple anti-hypertensive drugs. In today's world, we have little in terms of any pharmacologic treatment, other than control of high blood pressure to prevent hemorrhagic complications. Donepezil plays a little role in the management of this disease and was promptly removed from Pedro's care. We fortunately found a new home for him in an allied long-term care facility. Pedro waved and smiled toothily as he was wheeled out of our hospital.

It should not come as any surprise that as a prelude to Alzheimer's MCI carries the same unpredictable trait: it is austere or ductile, explicit or curtained, obedient or incoherent. The fact that it can serve as a preamble to several neurodegenerative dementias other than Alzheimer's, as well as to non-neurodegenerative conditions, like depression or medicine effects, makes it a very unpredictable entity. MCI exists only when we have definitive evidence of it. And if MCI has to be related to Alzheimer's, we have no option but to turn to the diagnostic tests that define Alzheimer's.

Where do we stand, then, in detecting MCI? For years, scientists, from molecular biologists to neurochemists, have been straining to detect any biomarker that may be associated with this disease.

Nearly twenty-five years ago, light was cast from across the Atlantic when scientist M. Vandermereen and his colleagues from the University of Antwerp's Laboratory of Neurobiology, Born-Bunge Foundation, detected in cerebrospinal fluid (CSF) an abnormal form of a protein, called tau, which is typically found in autopsies of Alzheimer's patients.

When structurally normal, it plays a pivotal role in the assembly of a microtubule (a ubiquitous structure responsible for cell division and movement) and the stability of our nerves. From some voiceless signal, this abnormal form of protein occupies the microtubules, rendering them useless with inevitable deleterious effects on the nerves.

As more research followed and more biomarkers poured in, a certain class of peptides comprised of forty-odd amino acids, called beta-amyloid, stole the limelight. What started off as a gentle curiosity soon became an obsession. In desperate eagerness, researchers could unravel the inside of the tangles that clogged an Alzheimer's brain. They learned that by forming plaques, these sticky beta amyloid clumps could block cell-to-cell signals and trigger immune system cells to create an inflammatory havoc that would completely disable the brain cells. A glimpse into the CSF to detect an unusually low number of beta-amyloids, and thereby large numbers trapped in the brain, soon became an objective marker to hunt down Alzheimer's.

Some of the best results came from genetic studies.

For the early onset Alzheimer's disease (EOAD), we have unraveled three known causative genes whose mutations have hastened the process: *PSEN1*, *PSEN2*, and *APP*. Scientists caution us, though, that when interpreting these test results, mutations have also shown variable expression, both within and between families.

A certain apolipoprotein gene (APOE) has been identified and linked to late onset Alzheimer's disease (LOAD). Functionally, these genes help in the synthesis of apolipoprotein E, which, as a carrier of cholesterol, helps in amyloid aggregation and clearance of the deposits from the brain. Understandably, in the absence of this gene, excessive beta amyloid deposits in the brain, which, as we know, forms the landmark findings in Alzheimer's patients. A specific form (also termed alleles) of this gene is of particular interest to us. Called APOE ε4, this allele is present in about 25 to 30 percent of the population and in about 40 percent of all people with late onset Alzheimer's disease. In other words, people who develop Alzheimer's disease are more likely to have an APOE ε4 allele than people who do not develop the disease.

Appropriately, APOE ε4 is looked upon as a risk factor gene because it increases a person's risk of developing the disease. However, true to the vagaries of this disease, it has also been shown that just the inheritance of an APOE ε4 allele will not conclusively drive an individual to Alzheimer's disease. This means that although a blood test can identify which APOE alleles a person has, it cannot predict by any means who will or will not develop Alzheimer's.

As a result, we seem to fall back into the same bottomless dungeon with beautiful findings containing little specificity or sensitivity. As of now, most researchers preach that this APOE ε4 gene can be used to study the risk of developing the disease in a large cohort of people—something like mass or herd testing—but not for determining any one person's risk. This conundrum has triggered intense debates as to whether individuals should be tested at all for a disease that has no clear cure on the approaching horizon. The necessary fear is that, if tested positive, but with a guarantee of its predicting value, it will only introduce anxiety, apprehension, and depression, all of which are capable of negatively affecting one's psyche.

All of these stem from a direct-to-consumer (DTC) genetic testing company, 23andMe, that introduced the testing as an option for customers of European ancestry. Accordingly, customers who have been genotyped on the company's latest platform—or who are willing to upgrade—can choose to learn whether they carry the disturbing APOE ε4 gene.

Muin Khoury, director of the Centers for Disease Control's (CDC) Office of Public Health Genomics, and a big opponent of the gene test, has advised that in the wake of an insufficient level of demonstrated clinical utility, APOE testing "should be offered in a medical setting, with counseling," and should not be made available DTC. Similarly, in the fall of 2010, the European Society of Human Genetics issued guidelines opposing "the premature DTC commercialization of various genetic tests," including tests for which clinical utility is unproven. Soon after, researchers from Boston University conducted the Risk Evaluation and Education for Alzheimer's (REVEAL) disease study. This study showed that the test "did not result in significant short-term psychological risks." The researchers emphatically added that after the initial disclosure of APOE status, "test recipients still consider[ed] the pros to strongly outweigh the cons."

The hunt for a target marker continues. In a recent study from Temple University's Department of Pharmacology and Center for Translational Medicine, scientists starved mice brains of glucose and found that the deficit promoted high levels of phosphorylated tau, mediated by the activation of a protein pathway, called P38 MAPK Kinase. Published in the 2017 *Journal of Translation Psychiatry*, the article pinned hope on p38 as a possible candidate for a novel drug development.

In the meantime, so as not to fall behind, neuroimaging jumped into the fray. In 2012, the U.S. Food and Drug Administration approved the first molecular imaging tracer for use with patients being evaluated for possible Alzheimer's disease or other causes of cognitive decline. This tracer (brand name Amyvid, but also known as florbetapir F-18) is a molecule that binds to beta-amyloid in the brain. Because it is labeled with a radioactive tracer, it can be visualized during a positron emission tomography (PET) brain scan, thereby revealing the presence of amyloid plaques in the brains of living patients.

The following year brought Vizamyl, known as flutametamol F18, which also binds to and reveals amyloid plaques in the brain during PET imaging. A third molecular imaging tracer (brand name Neuraceq, but known as florbetaben F18) was approved in 2014, and like its two predecessors, binds to and reveals amyloid plaques in the brain during PET imaging.

Close on the heels of all these neuroimaging ventures came a functional version—Pittsburgh compound B (PIB), nicknamed after its founder, the University of Pittsburgh, as the first radiotracer capable of highlighting deposits of beta-amyloid. Within a year, Florbetaben

(BAY 94-9172) arrived, another radiotracer designed to detect beta-amyloid during a PET scan.

But before the scientific fraternity could break into rapturous celebration, it was learned that these amyloid plaques were neither sensitive nor specific for Alzheimer's. In fact, they could be present even in normal, healthy individuals who show no cognitive decline. As recently as 2016, Dr. Nunzio Pomara, Professor from the Department of Psychiatry at New York School of Medicine, learned that major depression might lead to elevations of the potentially neurotoxic Amyloid Beta Species that is *independent* of Alzheimer's disease.

This supposed progress brings us back to exactly where we started centuries ago with a physician's eyes, ears, and fingers on a patient's pulse, exhibiting the priceless commodities of a healer. We need these practitioners as desperately as we need imaging studies and disease markers. While the world struggles to attain the latest and best innovations, it will do us good as providers to return to, and preserve, the elemental and the natural.

The Mini Mental Status Examination (MMSE), the Montreal Cognitive Assessment, (MoCA), Sweet 16 (an open-access brief cognitive screening instrument), Addenbrooke's Cognitive Examination (ACE), and the Saint Louis Mental Status Examination (SLUMS) are all expressions of patient-doctor interactions, tools to help doctors reach out to patients. They are all sets of questionnaires, among which lies the diagnosis of a mind beginning to falter, unmasking a seed of devastation beyond measure.

2

DRUGS, DRUGS, DRUGS: MODERN MEDICINE'S COMMODITY FETISHISM

I don't do drugs. I am drugs.

—Salvador Dali

Coming from a physician who encourages and endorses the appropriate use of over-the-counter drugs and routinely prescribes FDA-approved medications, including controlled substances, this chapter may appear paradoxical. To the millions who otherwise would have been crushed under the boots of infectious and noninfectious diseases, this might even seem blasphemous. It is not my intention to castigate the same drugs, which human lives and my academic expertise depend on. Neither should the following pages be viewed as the retreating steps of a physician close to retirement from active practice. I am not a leader of a vanguard or a whistle blower.

For the last thirty years, I have practiced clinical medicine, which rests on a triad of diagnosis, treatment, and prevention, and prescription and nonprescription drugs are legitimate and undisputed fulcrums of many cures. Yet from this very throne of power brews a resistance in the making, and like a landmine at every bend, this resistance stems from the way we practice care today.

To be specific, the insurmountable challenge comes from the *overuse* of drugs. Like any human trait that is indulged once it promises and promotes happiness, we, too, overexercise our power to control and conquer. And like any power-hungry souls, we bleed from the very sword we create to protect and preserve. We will go down the memory lane to witness the highs and lows of our battle with drugs that has led us to our present field of conflict. History will explain our present and hopefully guide our future.

In the making of today's pharmaceutical industry, one word has played a sterling role. Its eleven letters conspired in hushed creativity and plotted medical history's most telling concept. Simply called "serendipity," this word spins out of Serendip, an old Arabic name for Ceylon, presently referred to as Sri Lanka. Its origin, however, is from a Persian fairy tale where the Three Princes of Serendip were "always making discoveries, by accidents and sagacity, of things they were not in quest of." The tale travelled from Persia to Italy to France, until it fell into the hands of Horace Walpole, an English man of letters who chiseled out a new English word in a letter to his friend, Horace Mann, in 1754. Thus was born *serendipity*.

Every modern English discovery shares the same feeling for serendipity. It is either "the faculty of making happy and unexpected discoveries by accidents" (*Oxford English Dictionary*) or "the faculty of finding valuable or agreeable things not sought for" (*Webster's*). As would be expected, in the world of drug-seeking medicine, serendipity implies the finding of one thing while searching for another.

As history would have it, twelve drugs by sheer chance came out of nowhere to become pioneers in patient care. Like twelve disciples, they surrounded the holy and went on to permeate major disease states that have continually tormented human minds and bodies.

As Louis Pasteur famously wrote, *"Dans les champs de l'observation, le hazard ne favorise que les espirits prepares"* or, in short, "Chance favors the prepared mind." As would be expected, the twelve drugs did not have the same birth dates, although they were huddled around the same time periods. Six were found while the founders were looking for something else: aniline purple, penicillin, lysergic acid diethylamide, meprobamate, chlorpromazine, and imipramine. In the birth of three drugs—potassium bromide, chloral hydrate, and lithium—an abjectly wrong rationale gave way to an accidentally correct empirical result. Iproniazid and sildenafil became indications of diseases that were not even known. The remaining chlordiazepoxide came out of pure luck, discovered during a laboratory cleanup.

It all started in 1856, when William Henry Perkins, an eighteen-year-old English chemist, while trying to synthesize quinine, ended up creating a "black mess" in his test tube that he later realized had excellent dyeing qualities. Variously called niline purple, tyrian blue, or mauve, his discovery of an artificial dye paved the way for some of the greatest dye industries of the world: Bayer (1862), Ciba (1859), Geigy (1859), and Sandoz (1862). A new branch of science called organic chemistry became a necessary advancement, and inevitably, as if ordained by the almighty, all those dye industries became houses of organic compounds. The saga of the pharmaceutical industry started soon after, with Bayer and Ciba leading the way.

Accidental Penicillin

Being the king of all drugs, let me single out penicillin and its war path, as it evolved over the years. Most inventions—noble, profound, and groundbreaking—have gushed from inspirations, sudden and exotic. A freakish thought, like a streak of lightning, can blind the earth and take the world by storm. From Newton's apple to Edison's bulb, new concepts have struck quickly and suddenly rather than tenuously and tediously. But never has history witnessed such a life-changing invention springing out of sheer negligence.

We move to 1928 and the lab of Alexander Fleming in the basement of St. Mary's Hospital in London, now part of Imperial College. One day, while hustling out of his lab, Fleming, an otherwise fastidious and brilliant Scottish scientist, must have been rather slapdash in the proper placement of his Petri dishes that were growing staphylococcus bacteria. This oversight allowed a number of opportunistic molds from an open window to invade the cultured colonies. When Fleming returned the following day, he found to his giddy delight that half of the colonies had been cleaned up by these blue-green invaders. He studied the chemical and made one of the greatest discoveries of the modern world—penicillin.

Fleming published all his results in the *Journal of Experimental Pathology* in 1929. Unfortunately, it was a full decade before Howard Florey and his team could develop a sophisticated methodology to extract and eventually produce penicillin. Two years later, John Mahoney and his colleagues in the U.S. Public Health Service gave the world the best news it might have heard in a long time. They demonstrated that penicillin could be used to treat syphilis. There must have been wild jubilation across the globe, as few had been spared from the wrath of syphilis.

For the next few decades, penicillin ruled the world. Sweeping through world wars and cold wars and the strains and stains of all of them, the original antibiotic and its synthetic forms fought endless battles. From neurosyphilis to a sore throat, penicillin was a charmer that swayed the snake at will.

Let's move on and take the example of a non-antibiotic. In 1945, meprobamate came out of London's British Drug Houses Ltd. as an effective antimicrobiological agent. However, during his research, Frank Berger noticed that when it was given to mice, rats, or guinea pigs, they all happily dozed off, momentarily, but effectively. Berger crossed the Atlantic, joined hands with Wallace Laboratories, and soon meprobamate rolled out as the world's leading anti-anxiety agent. Wallace Laboratories called it Milltown, the name of a small community in New Jersey where Berger lived and worked.

By the late 1950s, meprobamate had emerged as the world's leading anti-anxiety prescription drug. For a decade it went unchallenged, until diazepam came on the scene and put an end to its dynasty. In capsule, tablet, and elixir forms, similar to meprobamate, diazepam found a home in every nook and corner of the human body.

A drug-churning world never looked back. Like Caesar and his armies, these drugs came, saw, and conquered. Miracle after miracle followed. Industry-endorsed compounds resulting from countless trials roamed unchallenged under the patronage of existing governments.

Resistance:
The Scourge of Every Drug Born

Caught in the deafening din of success, science failed to hear the silent steps of an ambush. It had blindly trusted the chemicals it had created. The power of those compounds was all that mattered to the scientific vision, not the power of the vanquished. At that time, biology had little knowledge of the boundless capabilities of genes, of their omnipresence and omnipotence, as well as their ability to recover *and* resist. A new world order would be formed, one encompassing cure and resistance, walking hand in hand.

As would be expected, penicillin became one of the major drugs to initiate this spectacle. In their zeal for the absolute cure, and with scarce knowledge of how bacteria can behave, most clinicians prescribed penicillin for just about anything to nearly anyone. From syphilis to a sore throat to any assumed superimposed bacterial infections, the drug became the panacea of all cures. However, it took time for scientists to visualize and reveal the complex structure of this relatively simple molecule.

In 1949, British biochemist Dorothy Crowfoot Hodgkin revealed a clue through her X-ray crystallographic studies. It would take the scientific fraternity another ten years before John Clark Sheehan, an American organic chemist, would perform the "the first rational synthesis of a natural penicillin." But by this time, the drug had been out in the market, which meant that resistant strains of bacteria capable of inactivating the drug were equally rampant. The war bugle had been sounded, and there would be no retreat.

An even more deeply disturbing event surfaced during those tumultuous times. In 1940, twelve years after Alexander Fleming discovered penicillin and several years before the drug actually got marketed, Edward Penley Abraham, a British biochemist and Oxford University professor, spearheaded the discovery of bacterial penicillinase. This enzyme could effectively cleave the beta lactam ring, considered the backbone of the drug.

Almost like a death sentence, the following information had to be faced: a large number of antibiotic r genes (resistance genes) are actually components of our natural microbial populations. Suddenly, scientists were facing the most difficult question ever asked: Which came first, the antibiotic or the resistance?

With no answer on the near horizon, the eye-for-an-eye battle started. Scientists performed studies to chemically modify penicillin so as to prevent cleavage. Several synthetic versions of the natural penicillin followed. Bacteria hit back with characteristic ferocity. Methicillin Resistant Staphylococcus Aureus (MRSA), Vancomycin Resistant Enterococci (VRE), Extended Spectrum Beta Lactamase (ESBL), all became fearful names to be held in awe.

All other antimicrobials met identical fates. Sulfonamides, introduced in 1937, produced resistant strains. Then came streptomycin in 1944. The drug was heralded as lifesaving in its management of tuberculosis. Until then, *Mycobacterium Tuberculosis* had behaved like a serial killer, gunning down men, women, and children with no rhyme or reason. Fear became the primary emotion whenever anyone coughed.

The words of Victorian poet John Keats highlight the agony and terror of tuberculosis. On February 3, 1820, Keats had returned from London to his New Hampstead house shivering in fever. As Charles Brown, his very close friend, wrote, "He mildly and instantly yielded to my request that he should go to bed. . . . On entering the cold sheets, he slightly coughed. And I heard him say, 'That is blood in my mouth. . . . I know the color of that blood; it is arterial blood . . . that drop of blood is my death warrant; I must die.'"

Streptomycin put on the brakes, but ever so slightly. Mutant strains of *Mycobacterium tuberculosis* resistant to therapeutic concentrations of the antibiotic surfaced quite soon during patient treatment. In 1946, the Medical Research Council (MRC) TB unit in the United Kingdom conducted the first documented randomized, controlled clinical trial where Streptomycin, along with bed rest, was compared with only bed rest. The trial showed that although the combination approach achieved greater clinical efficacy, the pathological improvement was marginal.

Eight years later, in 1952, a team of medical researchers from Cornell Medical College learned that tuberculosis raged untreated on a Navajo Reservation in Arizona. These researchers, led by Walsh

McDermott, saw a golden opportunity to feed on the ill health of a marginalized population. They started a ten-year project to evaluate the efficacy of new antibiotics. It also unveiled the bitter side of human research—the power and reach of modern medicine to experiment on an impoverished population in the name of advancement. Nevertheless, Isoniazid (INH), as an anti-TB drug, was soon manufactured. Patients fared far better with the two-drug approach of Streptomycin and INH. But sure enough, resistance emerged. Scientists prowled for another antibiotic. Rifampicin came along in the 1960s as a major breakthrough. For the first time, we started to save lives from TB. The U.S. Public Health Services joined hands with the United Kingdom's MRC TB unit, and over the next four decades, intense research produced two more drugs—pyrazinamide and ethambutol—that along with INH and rifampicin made a four-drug regimen that finally seemed like it could harness the bacteria.

But by then, the more medications scientists piled into the world, the more furious came the resistance. The cocktail of anti-TB drugs could stall the death-killing spree, but resistance refused to surrender. Newer terminologies to comprehend the unending appetite of resistant TB strains have emerged in recent years, including Extremely Drug-Resistant (XDR) strains, and then Totally Drug Resistant (TDR) strains. A firm verdict emerged: antibiotic resistance in TB occurs exclusively by spontaneous mutation.

In Mycobacterium *leprae*, we had merciless bacteria. While mycobacterium *tuberculosis* had a knack for killing people, Mycobacterium *leprae* pleasured in disfiguring people. They chose nerves as their favored place of residence and streamed through the body in endless colonies. They particularly aimed for the finest, peripheral nerves that control the various muscles. Mycobacterium *Leprae* simply froze the internal ropes of a human being. One by one, the muscles became affected, giving rise to both wasting and weakness. The sensory system was damaged, and ulcers and infections entered the body at will. Amputations became common.

A clueless medical fraternity made up new names for these victims: lepers or leonine facies, among terrible others. History would provide great examples of benevolence from churches and private organizations. However, these victims were generally shunned by the world. These "different-looking" men and women colonized in caves, gutters, and wherever darkness shielded them, waiting for some divine inspiration to heal them.

From the early 1900s through the late 1940s, doctors in Africa, Asia, the Far East, South America, and elsewhere injected leprosy patients with chaulmoogra oil. This oil has long been used in India as Ayurvedic medicine for the treatment of leprosy and various skin conditions. While historical anecdotes provide evidence of its scattered benefits, research was inconclusive.

The suffering and isolation continued unabated until Promin, a sulfone drug, arrived in 1937. As we now know, credit for bringing this drug to earth actually goes to Emil Fromm, professor of chemistry in the medical faculty of the University of Freiburg im Breisgau in Germany, who described this compound related to the sulphonamides: diaminodiphenylsulphone or dapsone (DDS).

Dapsone soon replaced the crude chaulmoogra oil and the world erupted in joy and relief. "Lepers" returned to their communities. Skin spots faded. Nerves were protected. Muscles were intact. Wounds were healed. But the scars remained. The stigma of being a leper would never disappear and pervaded all nuanced understanding. Leprosy as an infectious disease continued, hushed and hidden.

Within the next decade or so, scientists sadly realized that the world's only treatment for this ruthless disease was rendered useless by a resistant form of the mycobacterium. Across the globe, scientists pushed the limits for the next generation of effective drugs.

Clofazimine and rifampicin were discovered in the 1960s and 70s. These, along with Dapsone, finally became the three-drug regimen to kill this ravenous organism.

Despite the spate of success with mycobacterium and others, scientist were forever vexed by one disturbing verdict passed down by the Japanese in the 1950s: that antibiotic resistance could be genetically transferred and disseminated globally among all bacterial colonies. Subsequent discoveries that antibiotics were not just for killing bacteria, but could also be used as antiviral, antitumor or anticancer agents, completed the cyclone of sorrow. Resistance was no more the sole prerogative of infectious diseases. Genes would take us to a different level of understanding medicine—a sublime crossroad of universality and individuality—detachment and attachment at the same time, as one brilliant drug provided fresh fodder for another brilliant form of *resistance.*

Psychiatry's Rocky Voyage

The advent of psychiatry as a rigid subspecialty came about reluctantly, a forced result of an aberration that society was not happy to handle. In the early nineteenth century, asylums and hospitals were packed with "lunatics" and "abhorred" men and women who were "condemned" for being born differently. They did not incite scientific interest or invention, as did the flu, or malaria, or even syphilis. The term *psychiatry* was born at this time, even though there were no psychiatrists to handle these matters. Instead, mental illness was considered a nerve-related issue, and neurologists looked nervously at behavior that was termed *neurotic.*

One Austrian neurologist, Sigmund Freud, decided to dive into the unseen cloud of the human mind. His theories, what he called the "royal road to the unconscious," delved deeply into the unconscious roots of mental anomalies, which became formally known as psychoneurosis. Obsessed with the hidden and the surreal, Freud led the way, from the 1890s onwards, in the "medical" management of psychiatric disorders, ranging from hysteria to mutism.

Psychoanalysis as a major treatment module was born from these roots and has stood the test of time and the onslaught of pharmaceutical industries. In those early days, it suffered from a lack of any formal school of thought and training. As a result, it underachieved and overreacted randomly, paving the way for other interventions.

One such intervention was known as the icepick method, a practice that began in the 1940s and prevailed for the next two decades. It has since been variously called crude and illegal. Walter Freeman II was the founder, pioneer, and proponent of this much-maligned intervention, also known as a lobotomy.. The concept was not exactly his brainchild. In fact, Portugese neurologist Egas Moniz was drilling skulls to treat mental patients in a procedure called a leucotomy. Freeman imbibed the idea, made it gentler, and renamed it lobotomy. It entailed inserting a tool similar to an ice pick beneath the eyelid into the brain through the thin bone of the eye socket, and fiddling with the neural fibers in the hope of resetting normalcy.

In the early 1940s and 1950s, with no serious therapeutic cure, the practice flourished and was considered revolutionary. William Laurence, a reporter from *The New York Times*, lauded it as a "surgery for the soul." A staggering 40,000 Americans underwent this procedure, peaking at 5,000 annually in 1949. It became so popular and fashionable at the time that hundreds of people volunteered to procure surgical tools to be inserted into their brains—twice—and some as many as three times.

A sprinkling of successes was overshadowed by famous failures, and the practice ended when a patient seeking her third lobotomy, Helen Mortensen, died on the operating table in 1967. Soon after, Dr. Freeman was stripped of his medical license.

Was it insanity or desperation that drove Dr. Freeman to invent such a method?

I posed this question to his son, and Berkeley neurologist, Dr. Walter Freeman III, whose answer was quick and emphatic.

"Desperation. People forget in what deplorable state psychiatric patients lived and survived in those asylums during those days. Anything and everything had to be attempted to relieve them from their grotesque state of being."

Before the Second World War, more than 400,000 Americans lived in 477 asylums, and psychiatric patients occupied half of those beds. Dr. Freeman opined that his father was doing what was best for his patients, performing lobotomies for a meager $25 for those in the most desperate and impoverished circumstances.

The Decade of the Brain

Drugs finally came to the rescue in the 1950s. Thorazine, along with the first generation of antipsychotic drugs, completely changed the face of psychiatry with the same melodramatic effects that Levadopa-Carbidopa had on patients stifled with Parkinson's disease in the 1960s. The "de-institutionalization movement" must have been one of the most gratifying moments in medical history. The doors of asylums and hospitals were flung open as "lunatics" with firm diagnoses of psychotic disorders reentered society as human beings, protected by prescriptions, just like any other diseased individual.

What followed was profuse and almost justifiable. Psychoanalysis and psychodynamics were swept aside as unscientific and adolescent. Pharmaceutical companies tasted blood as new classes of antidepressants, called SSRIs (Selective Serotonin Reuptake Inhibitors) and new antipsychotics, called atypical neuroleptics, with blatant and superior qualities, flooded the marketplace. Prescriptions flowed—not just from psychiatrists but from primary care and family physicians. The National Institute of Mental Health dubbed the 1990s the Decade of the Brain.

Not to be left behind, clinical psychologists joined the fray with their arsenal of cognitive behavioral psychotherapies. Termed Cognitive Behavioral Therapy (CBT), it quickly and eagerly followed the same cow path of drugs: relief of symptoms. This method, along with the drugs, held the reins together for many years.

The pattern was unmistakable. They staged emotional quotients, compartmentalizing each other under firm diagnosis, and set about curbing specific symptoms by defining the diagnosis. No one doubted their success. Lunatics condemned to asylums were finally transformed into healthy human beings capable of normal lives.

But soon after it became clear that mere alleviation of the symptoms was not akin to a cure. Bipolar remained bipolar, and schizoid remained schizoid in muffled states and hiding. Depression lurked beneath the gloss, despite mood elevation. More important, previously unknown adverse effects—some subtle and some dramatic—surged. Serotonin Syndrome, secondary to SSRIs and Neuroleptic Malignant Syndrome, became fearful complications, presenting with hyperthermia, confusion, and other neurological symptoms.

In certain instances, people taking SSRIs reported increased suicidal tendencies. To make matters worse, these drugs had to be taken for the duration of one's life. The slightest disobedience gave rise to "discontinuation syndromes," with frightful symptoms of renewed depression, hostility, and agitation. As if this was not enough, at a more fundamental level and despite lavish financial contributions to pharmaceutical companies, newer discoveries completely dried up. Scientists stumbled beyond neurotransmitters.

As the year 2005 came to a close, scientists and scholars gathered for a symposium called *Advances in Neuroscience for Medical*

Innovation (ANMI). They hailed from all branches and sub-branches of neuroscience, including stress, memory, molecular pharmacology, animal behavior, pharmacogenetics, imaging, and drug discovery and development.

Unlike other symposia held around the world, this one, in a remarkable display of self-contemplation, took a completely different route by putting the experts on the spot. The symposium centered on five fundamental challenges facing them and their specialized societies. Expert voices were heard, some discerning, some lamenting, some critical, but all harmonious in one single clarion tone, exclaiming that the light at the end of the tunnel exists in a better integration of molecular, cellular, and system-level knowledge of psychiatric disorders.

The first of the five questions shot out like a bullet to the head:

> *Why have efforts in the discovery of new drugs for psychiatric disorders been relatively unsuccessful compared with other disease areas?*

With closer attention to the tone of the question, one might feel the strain of psychiatry. Unlike bludgeoning advances made in other departments, including cancer and disorders of the heart, the field of psychiatry, despite generating life-changing drugs, has suffered immensely because of the modern concept of medical management—despite the resurgence of Clozapine (*atypical* antipsychotic used for schizophrenia) at the turn of the twenty-first century after being dumped in Europe in the 1970s and Prozac appearing as "a breakthrough drug for depression" on the front cover of *Newsweek* in March, 1990.

More questions confronted the field of psychiatry.

> *Why do some minds with identical, mirror-like disorders respond while others do not?*

Why do some diseases march on untouched by the ravages of time
while others get castrated midway?
Why do psychiatric drugs continue to explode and implode with
no sense of democracy or decency when it comes to the failing
human mind?

Answers that came from the invited experts at the symposium carried the astonishing alacrity and honesty of a fraternity that has been increasingly troubled in its inability to fathom a brain that, as an organ, seemed far more intricate and skewed than the experts ever thought.

In general, life-shaping discoveries have sprung from gory experiments where rats were given cancers, mice hearts were tampered with, while others got inoculated with chemical compounds introducing one disease after another.

With the diseased mind, however, traditional scientific approaches were stopped in their tracks. How can you give depression to a mouse? How can anxiety be introduced to an already anxious rat? How can you create a bipolar guinea pig or, more tantalizingly, stun the *animalish* brain into a state of Alzheimer's?

Scientists have been working on it. They have been working on both transgenic (where the original genome is modified by the insertion of a trans gene) and knock out (when a gene is deleted) mice. But the challenges have been huge with a clear lack of concordance between preclinical trials and human clinical trials.

Most experts agreed that psychiatric drugs suffered from a lack of animal models.

Far worse and more fundamentally, the diseases of the brain, be they grievous, hostile, unsure or devoid of memory, are completely heterogeneous and lacking in any conformity or discipline. As Dr. Husseini Manji, Global Therapeutic Head for Neuroscience at Janssen

Research and Development, and NIH's former Chief of the Laboratory of Molecular Pathophysiology and Experimental Therapeutics, put it, "The Diagnostic and Statistical Manual (DSM-IV) is based on the clusters of symptoms and characteristics of a clinical course that do not necessarily describe homogeneous disorders, but rather reflect final common pathways of different pathophysiological processes involving genetics and environmental contributions."

For example, while all livers are born equal and, when cirrhotic, exhibit near-identical tissue pathologies, brains are not functionally equal and their disease states do not represent a common pathology. Depression, as a manifestation of a multitude of symptoms with variability and response to various treatments, is a conglomeration of multiple disease states. We seldom confront depression or Alzheimer's or schizophrenia as a lonely wolf. These diseases may not always hunt in packs, but traces of each seem dragged along by the other.

A perfect example is that of Parkinson's and its flirtations with various types of dementia. Scientists have added a whole new spectrum of diseases called *Parkinson-Like Syndrome*, trying to place them under the same umbrella. While Parkinson's disease as the parent body exhibits the classical triad of resting tremor, bradykinesia (lack of ancillary movement), and rigidity, the *Plus Syndromes* are weighed down by motor weakness, instability, and dementia, often lacking *tremor*—the trademark feature of its ancestor.

In fact, Parkinson's tryst with Alzheimer's was a forgone conclusion, based on its ever-expansive repertoire.

This means that the chance of finding a tissue diagnosis in any given disease of the mind is more remote than finding a needle in a haystack. The bottom line remains, as David Diamond pointed out, that by and large all diseases of the mind can only be diagnosed subjectively through behavioral tests, as opposed to markers or reports, which are hopelessly lacking in these cases.

The much-talked about and researched receptor-ligand interactions where drugs target neurotransmitters for mood elevations (such as with Prozac and Cymbalta) have been the pharmaceutical industry's one single obsession for several decades, with little understanding and few attempts to explore other fields, like molecular pharmacology and biological psychiatry.

The inevitable result is a clutter of drugs aimed to curb signs and symptoms otherwise clueless to the dictations of an altered mind.

No one epitomizes the mayhem better than my father-in-law, Prasenjit Chaudhuri.

He possessed a keen intellect, ferociously read all that fell under his eyelashes, and reveled in arguments that leapt from philosophy to politics with a vivacious appetite. Health-wise, he lived a flawless life.

At the stroke of eighty, he noticed a slowing of his gait. It was more of a shuffle, he thought. In the ensuing weeks, he had difficulty raising himself from his chair. He needed someone to pull him up each time he attempted to stand. His gait became unsteady. He preferred short steps so as not to lean over. He felt weak and, in certain situations, even had a sense of freezing over. There was no tremor. The neurologist who examined him started him on Levadopa-carbidopa, the undisputed healer of Parkinson's disease.

With no improvement seen from the pills, he panicked. Melancholy settled in. He turned inward. Words became scarcer and scarcer. Enter a psychiatrist. A rushed Mini Mental examination gave him 20 out of a maximum 30. Diagnosed with "possible" Alzheimer's, donepezil was started, and, following close on its heels, an antidepressant. Nothing happened. He was estranged from the world. Another drug was prescribed, a benzodiazepine called lorazepam, to curb his growing anxiety.

Buffeted by quadruple "mind-curing" medications, Mr. Chaudhuri oscillated from tears to anger to nothingness. The doctor recommended an institutional approach. A new set of doctors arrived with fresh diagnoses and medications. Like new wine in an old bottle, some were withdrawn and some added. In a day or two, he started to hallucinate, first in bits and pieces, then in a continuous display of a fragmented mind, torn between images seen and imagined.

It became obvious that he was suffering from abrupt drug withdrawal. It was time to panic—this time for the doctors. They reintroduced lorazepam. Alzheimer's was not thought to be present. Donepezil was stopped. A touch of antidepressant remained.

An expressionless but stable Mr. Chaudhuri was sent home. He went back to what he always loved to do: meditation. According to him, this is how he gets his "peace of mind." He has recovered well since then. Till now, we do not have a firm diagnosis. The two remaining drugs have kept the symptoms down. I was delighted when he informed me that he was reading and enjoying *Hamlet* all over again.

Resistance and Diseases of the Mind

At this critical juncture, we turn our attention to Dr. Alison Little from the Oregon Health and Science University of Portland. Important yet disturbing statistics appeared in his study and analysis, published in *American Family Physician* in 2009.

Despite growing comprehension of this much-maligned disease of great longevity, only 60 percent of current patients in the United States with depression are actually subjected to treatment. Primary care physicians, very frequently the first and only doctors that patients see, detect depression in about one third or one half of their patients. When considering that the mean age of depression onset is as young as thirty, with a lifetime prevalence of 13 percent, one can only worry at the large percentage of missed diagnoses.

To complicate matters, despite the volume of antidepressants gushing from the pharmaceutical industry over the past twenty years, between one and two thirds of patients actually do not respond to the first line of prescribed antidepressants, and as high as 15 to 33 percent do not respond to subsequent interventions.

Schizophrenia offers the same disturbing research. Like depression, another nomenclature has been coined to adjust to the shifting paradigm of medical management: Treatment Resistant Schizophrenia (TRS). Why? The reasons are not difficult to guess. Much like depression, and despite appreciable advances in the therapeutics of schizophrenia, especially with the advent of Clozapine and other second-generation antipsychotics (SGAs), treatment-resistant schizophrenia continues to progress at a relentless rate.

Helio Elkis, MD, from Instituto de Psiquiatria HC-FMUSP, São Paulo, Brazil, and Peter F. Buckley, MD, from the Medical College of Georgia, delved into the depth of TRS. Published in the 2016 edition of *Psychiatric Clinical North American Journal*, their work highlighted the neurochemical mechanistic causes behind the emerging resistances, with particular emphasis on two neurotransmitters: dopamine and glutamine. Structural neuroimaging studies showed that patients with TRS exhibited a higher reduction of the prefrontal cortex volume, compared with non-TRS patients.

As would be expected, resistance, despite piling up added antipsychotics, has continued unabated. Is there hope? Authors have pinned their hopes on nonpharmacological strategies, such as transcranial magnetic stimulation or electroconvulsive therapy.

In a herculean effort to conquer the final frontier, scientists turned to genes to comprehend why some drugs achieve their desired effect while others do not. They unraveled mutation after mutation, trying to grasp the recalcitrant drugs. This approach was not entirely novel, given that mutations have been studied, used, and implicated in antibiotic and chemotherapy-resistant situations.

Called *pharmacogenomics*, the field quickly spread its wings over the victims of antidepressant and antipsychotic drugs. Simple saliva and blood tests could demonstrate and analyze various genes responsible for rendering resistance to specific drugs. The spectrum looked spectacular from a distance. Let us take a closer look.

SSRI Antidepressants
(Selective Serotonin Reuptake Inhibitors)

Examples

- Citalopram
- Flouxetine
- Paroxetene
- Sertraline
- Fluvoxamine

Genes Analyzed

- CYP2D6
- CYP3A4
- SLC6A4
- HTR2A

SNRI Antidepressants
(Selective Serotonin and Norepinephrine
Reuptake Inhibitors)

Examples

- Duloxetine
- Levomilnacipran
- Venlafaxine

Genes Analyzed

- CYP2D6
- CYP34A
- CYP2B6
- SLC6A4
- Benzodiazepines

Examples

- Clobazam
- Diazepam
- Alprazolam

Genes Analyzed

- CYP2C19
- CYP3A5
- Atypical Antipsychotics

Examples

- Clozapine
- Risperidone
- Olanzapine

Genes Analyzed

- CYP2D6

These charts have become commercially available. They are color-coded. The Green category indicates that the drug can be prescribed and used according to the FDA-approved drug label. The Orange category signals caution where the dosing levels need to be lowered or increased, or that the drug's side effects may cause an adverse reaction for the patient. The Red category indicates that the drug should be used with caution and with more frequent monitoring, due to the potential risk of a severe adverse reaction or lack of therapeutic response.

I will take only one of the above-mentioned genes to highlight the haze of the whole situation: CYP2D6.

As a member of the cytochrome P450 family of enzymes, CYP2D6 is involved in the oxidative metabolism of drugs. Being the most promiscuous of these enzymes, it displays large individual-to-individual variability in activity due to genetic polymorphisms.

How then does an individual respond to CYP2D6 activity when a drug is taken?

So far, we have been able to fathom four types: ultrarapid metabolizer (UM); extensive, or normal, metabolizer (EM); intermediate metabolizer (IM); and poor metabolizer (PM). To break it down further, if an individual is a UM, a drug taken would undergo an exaggerated pharmacological response, secondary to a very fast metabolism. Conversely, an IM or a PM would attenuate the effects of the drugs, as they are metabolizing at such a tedious rate. To make matters even more complex, the drugs themselves have variable impacts on CYP2D6, some being known to inhibit the very activity of the enzyme. For example, some of the drugs mentioned in the box, such as paroxetine, fluoxetine, and citalopram, are known to inhibit CYP2D6 activity and may actually convert EMs to IMs or PMs.

Imagine the chaos that will erupt when you bring in all the other genes, as shown in the chart, with their moods and tantrums specific to each individual.

In other words, no gene analysis is specific for any particular drug. An impossible number of overlapping genes with infinite permutations and combinations riddle the path toward any target. As genetic scientists continue usurping gene after gene, we wonder what this lead to and ask ourselves—*where does this end?*

Genetic mapping and sequencing have shattered age-old views of diseases. We have come to appreciate the foreplay and interplay between genes and environment. We now know that it's not the disease but an individual's unique genetic composition that will dictate the inception and prognosis of suffering. Like a disease, each drug's effect on an individual is solitary, with no comradeship.

For example, John's depression is different from Jill's depression, just as the effect of Prozac on John will be different from its effect on Jill. Call it the tip of an iceberg or the mouth of a volcano, but we are still leagues away from knowing what lies beneath the crust of our genetic existence.

Alzheimer's and Drugs:
The Ongoing Tragedy

Regarding Alzheimer's dementia, we are every bit like the five wise but blind men who are feeling different parts of an elephant and generating generous opinions of what it is. The diverse, and thoroughly unrelated theories about the genesis of Alzheimer's feel as discrete as the tusk, trunk, tail, teeth, and belly of the unseen animal. Among the countless theories trying to rationalize the aberration of the human mind, some verge on the romantic while others are worse than fanatic, but two theories stand out as plausible. They do not define the disease—far from it—but they do unearth fractions of milestones in the pathology of its events.

As scientists always do, they hunt for a counter-punch once a process is discovered. They blaze a trail as they follow the exact path of a disease process. From antihypertensive for high blood pressure to chemotherapy for cancer, this approach remains set in stone. This also applies to drugs for Alzheimer's. But given that the major road leading to Alzheimer's is yet undiscovered, no drugs can specifically blaze that trail.

We will start with cholinesterase inhibitors. Understanding that patients with Alzheimer's disease (AD) have reduced cerebral content of choline acetyl transferase (a transferase enzyme responsible for the synthesis of the neurotransmitter acetylcholine), there is a decrease in acetylcholine synthesis, which causes impaired cortical cholinergic function. This was thought to be one of the mechanisms underlying the functional wreck of the mind. True to the scientific spirit, scientists have engineered inhibitors of these neurotransmitters, based on the belief of increasing the much-needed cholinergic transmission in an environment defunct without the neurotransmitter.

Under the patronage of the pharmaceutical powerhouses, four cholinergic inhibitors rolled out. First came tacrine. Adrien Albert, a graduate from the University of Sydney, first used the drug as an antiseptic in 1940. William Summers used it in the 1970s on patients with drug overdose coma and delirium. He must have been influenced by Peter Davies, who was working in England on Alzheimer's disease. A decade later, from 1981 till 1986, Summers worked with Art Kling and his group at UCLA to demonstrate the usefulness of tacrine in Alzheimer's patients. The drug came into the market under the brand name of Cognex. Despite FDA approval, it died young, tossed out because of its ability to inflict severe hepatic toxicity (toxic effects on the liver) and other very serious gastrointestinal problems.

Pfizer, the multibillion-dollar company, then rolled out Donepezil. The drug was primarily researched at Esai, a Japanese pharmaceutical company headquartered in Tokyo, in 1983, under the supervision of Hachiro Sugimoto, a Japanese chemist and pharmacologist. In 1996, with FDA approval under its belt, Pfizer rolled it out as Aricept. The drug soon became the global star invading virtually every Alzheimer's mind with unrestricted entry. In an exciting 24-week double-blind study that entailed blinding both the examiners and the subjects of the study to be unaware of the drug being tested, significant improvement was seen, compared to the control groups, when measured by such standardized tests as the Alzheimer's Disease Assessment Scale, the cognitive subscale (ADAS-cog), and the Clinician's Global Impression of Change (CGIC). A euphoric world went forward with another trial. This time, it focused on 566 patients from memory clinics with mild to moderate AD. A small but significant beneficial effect of Donepezil or cognition compared with a placebo was observed with a 0.8 point difference in Mini Mental Status Exam (MMSE) scores.

The crash came soon after. Following the initial twenty-four-week study, researchers conducted the all-important six-week placebo washout study (the period allowed for all of the administered drugs to be eliminated from the body) to examine whether Donepezil had any disease-modifying activity. The results were horrific. The earlier improvements detected on cognitive measures had been completely erased, strongly suggesting that the drug did not affect the underlying course of the disease. Even worse, with no significant differences in global functioning, treatment-emergent adverse effects were more frequently observed in the higher-dose group. Nausea, vomiting, diarrhea, decreased heart rate, and, at times, brief unconsciousness, concluded this chapter of misery.

Undeterred, Novartis Pharmaceuticals manufactured Rivastigmine under the trade name of Exelon—another cholinesterase inhibitor, which was FDA-approved. Initially developed by Marta Weinstock-Rosin of the Department of Pharmacology at the Hebrew University of Jerusalem, the drug became available in liquid and capsule formulations in 1997. It demonstrated the same efficacies and adverse effects as its predecessor.

Scientists then tried something novel. In 2007, they manufactured a transdermal patch form of the drug to minimize the gastrointestinal side effects of nausea, vomiting, and diarrhea. Yet when it came to long-term benefits, the results were equally inconclusive.

Galantamine came next. FDA released it in 2001, nearly 50 years after Soviet pharmacologists M. D. Mashkovsky and R. P. Kruglikova-Lvova had worked on the drug's acetylcholine inhibitory properties. Previously called Reminyl and now Razadyne, the drug had similar effects but stole the limelight for a different reason. One particular study found that it actually increased mortality when given to patients with mild cognitive impairment.

With lesser adverse effects and comparable benefits, Donepezil emerged as the leading product, but nursing home patients who had advanced Alzheimer's dementia provided no conclusive data showing any comprehensive benefit. More important, for patients with mild cognitive impairment, considered possible precursors of Alzheimer's dementia, none of these drugs offered an olive branch.

Here lies the overarching tragedy.

Demonstrating short-term cognitive benefits without the power of prevention or cure, these drugs become a cruel tease for the sufferer. Yet, out of habit, and perhaps motivated by guilt, we continue to dispense these cholinesterase inhibitors.

With Memantine, scientists took another route. Glutamate was discovered as an excitatory amino acid found in the hippocampus area of the brain, the prime location for memory. It was found to activate a receptor, called NMDA, that is responsible for memory and learning. Because too much excitation is harmful to the nerves, the search was on to find an antagonist to oppose the excessive excitation. As an NMDA receptor antagonist, Memantine fit the bill perfectly. Haughtily termed a "neuroprotective" in the areas of memory and learning, it entered the market under the brand name Namenda.

This drug will also go down in history as another classic example of "serendipity." Before it was known as a neuroprotective agent, Memantine was touted as an antidiabetic agent and released into society by Eli Lilly and Company back in 1968. Found to be useless, it was sent back to the drawing board. More than twenty years later, the Merz Company from Germany found its neuroprotective effects and sent it back into circulation. This time, it was meant to save the brain from dementia. It took less than a decade for the U.S.-based Forest Company to shake hands with Merz, nickname it Namenda, and launch it into a society that was starving for another miracle drug.

Needless to say, Namenda did little to cure the demented brain. There was little, if any, evidence that patients with milder Alzheimer's dementia would benefit from this drug. Instead, a different set of adverse effects arose. With dizziness as its primary disturbing effect, the drug has been reported to cause confusion, hallucination, and, in some cases, agitation and delusional behaviors in patients with Alzheimer's dementia.

A 2008 systemic review by experts concluded that, "Memantine has been shown to improve cognition and global assessment of dementia, but with small effects that are not of clear clinical significance; improvement in quality of life and other domains are suggested but not proven."

Unanswered questions continued to pour in:

Will long-term treatment benefit those with mild AD?
Is it truly neuroprotective? How will that be manifested?
Will additional toxicities appear when it is used with larger numbers of people?

Almost all experts concurred that decisions to treat with Namenda are strictly to be determined on an individual basis, dependent on the physician, patient, or family choice, and must consider drug tolerability and cost. Unfortunately, this requires a perfect balancing act on a beam that does not actually exist.

In a market that is uncertain and volatile, it is natural to entertain all that a fertile mind can imagine. Endless cures and prevention strategies of Alzheimer's dementia scurry in and out like rats in an abandoned building. All have high convictions and minimum credibility. But they all are able to make noise, feeding on a society that is hapless and helpless in the grip of a disease that is determined to destroy our minds. It is futile and redundant to mention all these efforts. Instead, I will pick three of them as representatives, not because they were grand failures after heavily anticipated celebration, but because they highlight the audacity of their claims to fame.

Vitamin E and Selegiline

As a fat-soluble vitamin, an antioxidant, and an easy-to-access, attractive, over-the-counter medication, Vitamin E is an instant temptation. Firmly clinging to the belief that oxidative damage can hasten Alzheimer's disease, researchers from the Department of Neurology at Columbia University's College of Physicians and Surgeons, ran a double-blind, placebo-controlled, randomized, multicenter trial with patients with Alzheimer's disease of moderate severity. For two years, patients received Selegiline, believed to delay the disease process (essentially an anti-Parkinson's disease that can also be used as an antidepressant); alpha-tocopherol (Vitamin E, 2000 IU a day); both Selegiline and alpha-tocopherol, or a placebo. The scientists looked primarily for four outcomes:

+ Time taken to reach a combined endpoint of death,
+ Need for institutionalization,
+ Loss of ability to perform Activities for Daily Living (ADL), and
+ Progression to severe dementia based on a Clinical Dementia Rating scale.

A delayed progression to outcomes was noticed in the Vitamin E group and not in the Selegiline or placebo groups. However, a number of cognitive tests that were measured as secondary endpoints, including the MMSE and the Alzheimer's Disease Assessment Scale, cognitive subscale, failed to show any difference between the groups.

The numbers make for interesting reading that lead to assumptions that the researchers made that were, at best, preposterous, nervous, and desperate. The following numbers were shown to reflect delays in time to the primary outcome for the patients:

+ Selegiline (median time, 655 days),
+ Vitamin E (670 days),

+ Combination therapy of Vitamin E and Selegiline (585 days),
+ Placebo control group with no drug interventions (440 days).

Predictably, the researchers pointed out the 670 days of slower progression as being conclusive evidence of Vitamin E acting as a guardian angel for Alzheimer's patients. They were also happy that the Selegiline group did marginally better than the control group.

But when it came to the combination group, the researchers halted, stumbled, and completely somersaulted. If individually their champion drugs could slow progression, why did their combination (585 days) not produce an additive result? They were at a complete loss for words, as evident from the following statement:

> "There are several possible explanations for the lack of an additive effect of treatment. *Perhaps* both agents exert their effects through the same mechanism, with either agent providing a maximal benefit. Alternatively, each agent *may* work through an independent mechanism, but the disease may have been sufficiently severe that no additive benefit could be observed. Finally, one agent *may* interfere with the absorption or metabolism of the other, resulting in an effect that is not additive."

Regarding their *scientific* mechanism of action, the researchers remarked:

> "One can only *speculate* about the mechanism underlying this effect. Selegiline *may* have enhanced the functioning of nigral neurons or enhanced their survival by inhibiting oxidative deamination. Alpha-tocopherol *may* have provided the same benefit, resulting in the inability to observe an additive effect in the group receiving combined treatment."

The *New England Journal of Medicine*, considered the bible of all evidence-based resources, looked beyond the *mays* and *may nots*, went ahead and published the study.

Anti-inflammatory Drugs

Essentially "over-the-counter" painkillers, these are easily the weakest spot for the passersby striving for instant relief. Temptation comes from our conviction that all medical events happening around us are denouements of an inflammation. This leads to an inevitable generalization that anti-inflammatories can be used as life-savers for the Alzheimer's patients. From naproxen to aspirin, the shelves are full with these pretty bottles in various colors and shapes.

This time, Dutch scientists were tempted to step in. In the Rotterdam Study of 1998, from the Department of Epidemiology and Biostatistics, Erasmus University Medical School in the Netherlands, anecdotal reports indicated that the use of nonsteroidal, anti-inflammatory drugs (NSAIDs) may reduce the risk of Alzheimer's disease. Scientists studied the cross-sectional relation between NSAID use and risk for AD in a population-based study of disease and disability in older people.

Compared with all non-users, NSAID users had a lower risk for AD. Hope sprouted anew. Men and women began popping pain killers in their desire to kill arthritis and Alzheimer's with one swallow. However, the world soon realized that the Dutch work was essentially an epidemiological study, which warranted a clinical trial.

Four years down the road, out came a double-blind, placebo-controlled trial of diclofenac/misoprostol (an example of a non-steroidal and anti-inflammatory, MSAID) with mild to moderate Alzheimer's disease patients. This time Australian researchers from the Department of Clinical Pharmacology at St. Vincent's Hospital in Melbourne, ran this trial on 41 patients of mild-moderate AD in a prospective twenty-five-week trial. The trial showed an absolute opposite result. It did not demonstrate any significant effect of NSAID treatment in AD. Two years later, a second trial similarly nullified the Dutch study and virtually buried the analgesic fantasy. Anti-inflammatory drugs do not rejuvenate the dying mind. Worse, as an adverse effect, they can cause ulcers.

We stand today in a no-man's land, where overlapping diseases spew signs and symptoms for us to wash them away with buckets of pills. In between, patients remain inaccessible, captive in their own emotions.

Susan Perry comes to mind. While flipping through the chart of a newly established female patient, I gathered that she suffered from various psychiatric disorders. My nurse had all of my patient's morbidities dated to the month. However, what emerged from her detailed notes was strange and disturbing. This is what my patient's Past Medical History looked like:

Time of Onset	Diagnosis
December 2001:	Anxiety
July 2002:	Bipolar Disorder
September 2004:	Panic disorder
February 2006:	Major Depression, Borderline Personality Disorder

While hypothetically possible, did Susan really have all these emotional challenges? Who was making these diagnoses? Was it a solitary, over-exuberant psychiatrist, or had she shopped around for a bunch of internists and become callously labeled? Even more alarming was the endless list of medications she was subjected to. For each diagnosis, she was given an antidote: an anxiolytic, an antipsychotic, a sedative, and an antidepressant.

Although I was prepared to listen, Susan refused to talk to me. She was determined not to disengage herself from her silent, unspoken cocoon. All my open-ended questions remained unanswered.

"Would you like to share anything with me?"

"Do you have family support?"

"Do you need any counseling"?

Instead, Susan stood up abruptly and blurted out, "If you are not giving me the refills, I am getting out of here."

"I will continue some of the medications," I said, "but before that we need to . . ."

I started to reason with her but couldn't. She turned and stomped out in a flash.

Susan never came back. Three months later, she was brought to the emergency room with cardio-pulmonary arrest due to a possible heroin overdose. She died before she could be admitted.

MEDITATION: THE SCIENCE BEHIND AN ENDLESS ART

When faced with the vicissitudes of life,
one's mind remains unshaken, sorrow-less, stainless,
secure; this is the greatest welfare.

—Gautama Buddha

Roger Harper had a knack for numbers. As a corporate business executive, he had thrived on doing calculations in his head. But when he started struggling with familiar figures at age 63, he began to panic. His diminished abilities did not hit him overnight. At first, he thought it was the unending pressure of his job schedule and he took over-the-counter vitamins. The fumbling continued. Some days he was fluent. Some days he choked. Soon he was stressing, which made matters even worse. Someone in his office mentioned Alzheimer's disease.

When Roger came into my office, he was adamant about not taking any medication. He had read up on the subject, and he knew there was no cure. I did the Mini Mental on him. He actually passed with a good-looking score of 26. I assured him that he was not harboring any Alzheimer's Dementia. I reminded him about the necessity of being knowledgeable and to be cautious about the vagaries of this disease. He prided himself on his intelligence, and I realized from his demeanor that he was deeply disturbed. He wanted the fumbling to be fixed. But the very fact that he was not in denial gave me the opportunity to propose an alternative approach.

How about meditation?

I wasn't entirely surprised when Roger said he had heard about it before and had actually wanted to try it. He probably needed a physician like me to endorse the idea. I referred him to a certified instructor. For the past two years, Roger has been diligently practicing meditation. He still works in the same firm, feels much more in charge of his numbers, and excitedly reported an overall poise and confidence he had never felt before.

Catching Up to What I Already Knew

My knowledge of meditation is innate because I grew up surrounded by the ancient practice in India. Yet it did not seem to have much bearing on my knowledge and understanding of cognitive disorders until its effect on a friend of mine who began to suffer from Alzheimer's 20 years ago.

Many years my senior, Neel Roy, a high-ranking audit officer, had an endless repertoire of knowledge, ranging from classical music to politics. It came as a shock when he revealed that he was losing his memory. He seemed down and distraught, and by the time he told me, it was clear that this problem had been bothering him for quite some time.

"Are you forgetting familiar words?" I said.

I was a fresh out of medical school then and was going by the book.

He did not answer immediately. I let the silence linger until he was ready to say more. After a while he responded.

"I can't find the right words."

He was having trouble using the right words for the specific objects. For example, omelet, porridge, orange juice, and bread and butter got replaced by a universal term—breakfast. No one else noticed as it was a perfectly appropriate word. Though a chess player and a lover of philosophy, Roy was finding comfort in watching television, an act of comfortable surrender, where both his deficiency and dignity went untouched. He was sure he was coming down with Alzheimer's because it ran in his family.

That evening, I had little in terms of any tangible advice.

Check your thyroid

Give it some more time. You might be just anxious

Why don't you take an over the counter multivitamin?

Are you having trouble at home? At work?

He did not answer. It could have either have meant that those concerns or suggestions had already been entertained or he wasn't listening to me. Running out of options, I did what a just-born graduate would be inclined to do. I suggested a sub specialist. *A neurologist, maybe?*

Roy simply smiled and walked away.

I delved further into his issues. Spoke with seniors, flipped through pages, but made little headway. No diagnostic tests, no specific drugs. Literature was scant, ambiguous, and unsure. I was hitting a complete wall.

I called him up few days later.

"Why don't you try meditation?"

"Why?"

"Well, at worst, it is a relaxing exercise. At best, it is not a drug and has no side effects."

A month later, Roy was introduced to meditation through one of his friends. Following instructions, he took a candle to a quiet room. In an enchanted stillness, he sank into repeated cycles of meditation.

Today, 20 years later, Roy is approaching his 90s. He uses a walker, yet his brain is alert, awake, and as eager as a teenager's for what comes next.

I called him up from New York recently.

"So what's for breakfast?"

His reply came instantly.

"Milk and cereal, with a side of toast."

The Benefits of Calm

An extraordinary long-term study has been conducted since 1986 in Mankato, Minnesota. On Good Counsel Hill the convent of the School Sisters of Notre Dame sits in tranquil grandeur. In what is popularly called the Nun Study, the Catholic nuns have offered their genes for scientific analysis. They have been tested on various subjects, such as, how many words they can remember minutes after reading them on flashcards, how many animals they can name in a minute, and whether they can count coins correctly. They also wrote autobiographical essays when they first took their vows. When the nuns die, their brains are removed and shipped to a laboratory where they are analyzed.

The brilliance of this ongoing study lies in the similarity of its subjects. The nuns have identical living habits, precluding any environmental differences. None of them smoke, drink or become pregnant. They are all white females who attended good schools. More important, they all eat the same food from virtually the same cafeteria.

Published in *The Journal of Personality and Social Psychology*, an article about the study concluded that nuns who expressed more positive emotions in their autobiographies lived significantly longer—in some cases, ten years—than those expressing fewer positive emotions.

"I think the Nun Study is very important because it uses information obtained about people before the period of illness," says Dr. Robert P. Friedland, professor of neurology at Case Western Reserve University and the author of a study showing that people with Alzheimer's are, as young adults, less mentally and physically active outside their jobs than people without the disease. "So we know from the Nun Study and others that Alzheimer's disease takes several decades to develop, and the disease has many important effects on all aspects of a person's life."

Yet inevitable questions arise.

What exactly constitutes positive emotions?

"How much of this is temperament? How much of it is affected by life events and critical relationships with parents, friends, teachers, peers?" asked Dr. Richard Suzman, chief of demography and population epidemiology at the National Institute on Aging.

I will go a step further.

Are merely positive emotions the main protective factor against dementia?

We have already seen that a searching, intense mind does not guarantee safety from dementia. Dr. Bharati Sharma, a brilliant obstetrician and gynecologist, found herself drowned in abject dementia. Similarly, my grandmother, a scholar and a poet, wandered away and could not find her way back. Does the answer lie in a different direction entirely? We do not know the full truth yet. But it is becoming progressively apparent that stimulating mental challenges, such as solving crossword puzzles or reading tons of history books, do not necessarily prevent the onrush of dementia.

What is being found in test after test, is that meditation achieves much more than external focus. The benefits affect the deepest centers of the brain, causing structural and even functional changes that can effectively keep Alzheimer's at bay.

This is not just some feel-good vibe. It is a scientifically measured fact.

Meditation has come a long way since its primordial moments in the deep recesses of a forest, where ancient sages practiced this art as a way of life. From the teachings of Buddha to the research-laden laboratories of Ivy League institutes, it has taken a groundbreaking journey, offering one blessing after another. Scientific tests run by the Mayo Clinic, Johns Hopkins, and Harvard Medical School, among others across the globe, are both testimony and tribute to the endless potential of meditation.

As I have discussed, modern medical management adamantly follows strict, evidence-based findings. Nothing is considered standard unless it is held in our palms and felt. Any proposed advance must follow formal research protocols. A hypothesis is stated; the hypothetical drug and a placebo are given to "active" and "control" groups, respectively, and the results of each are compared. If tests show significant benefits reached through statistical analysis, the drug goes through further trials before being considered therapeutic.

Oddly enough, considering its philosophical origins, meditation has gone through identical research routes. The screaming headlines from various universities, much of which has been published in various journals, cannot be ignored. Meditation is being increasingly recognized as a powerful management tool for a variety of mental ailments. Specifically, it has emerged as a comprehensive therapy for minds affected by stress, depression, loss of memory, and other behavioral disorders.

Before we go too far, though, let us ask a very basic question: What is meditation?

Swami Vivekananda, considered the pioneer in preaching about and spreading meditation and yoga in the West, declared during a lecture in Chicago in 1893 that meditation was "the highest state of being."

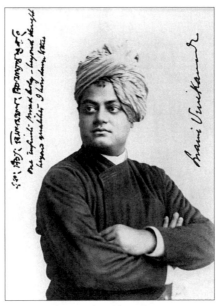

Swami Vivekananda in Chicago

While neuroscientists might smirk at this generalized opinion, more pragmatic clinicians have embraced meditation in a broad variety of practices. These range from techniques designed to promote relaxation to exercises performed to reach a heightened sense of well-being.

Despite changing names and perspectives passing down through the ages, two basic types of meditation have always led the way: open and focused. Mindfulness meditation is the open type, and transcendental meditation is the focused form. In simple terms, Open Monitoring (OM) meditation involves a relaxed, nonjudgmental awareness of the moment. Focused Attention (FA) meditation, by

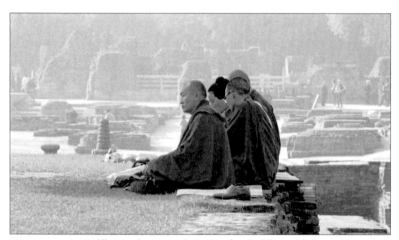

Buddhist monks at Sarnath, the city where Buddha preached.

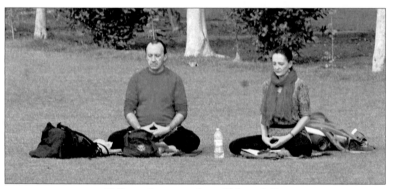

Meditators from across the world, Sarnath City.

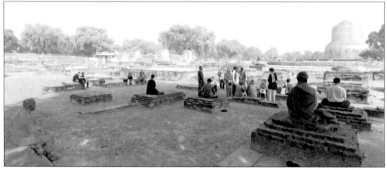

The Dhamekh Stupa in the Deer Park, Varanasi, Sarnath.

contrast, entails focusing attention on a chosen object in a continued, persistent fashion.

Both types have been the subjects of intense clinical study. One of the most researched meditation techniques is based on the concept of mindfulness. Traditionally based on the Buddhist practice, it focuses on breath and physical awareness with a goal to perceive without any judgment the thoughts that clutter our minds. Mindfulness in particular allows a person to stay "above" the tides of emotions that we feel every day. By conscious practice, your mind is trained to avoid falling into your usual, self-destructive behavioral patterns.

Let's take a look at the concepts, philosophies, and benefits of each type as they apply to minds in need of help and guidance.

Mindfulness Meditation: The Philosophy Behind It

To break apart the phrase *mindfulness meditation* in an attempt to seek the meaning of the individual words is like breaking one's spinal cord, which is at once fluent and continuous. The ease with which mindfulness weds meditation is a reflection of the profundity of the phrase. It is a tribute to the limitless gamut of its presence.

To the mind, however, in order to be felt in unison the two words need to be understood individually.

What, then, is mindfulness?

Very often, translation weakens the original. Every monumental piece of work, every sublime slice of a short story suffers each time the language changes. Be it Tagore, Maupassant, or Tolstoy, that "thing of beauty" fades a wee bit every time the primary source of expression is replaced. Yet translation is the only way words can travel. Otherwise, Tagore would remain in Shantiniketan, Maupassant in Tourville-sur-Arques, and Tolstoy in the Tula province of Russia. To the

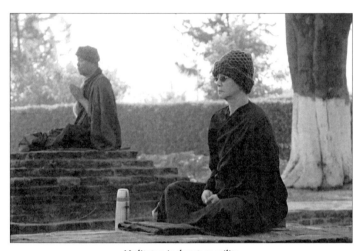

Meditators in deep tranquility.

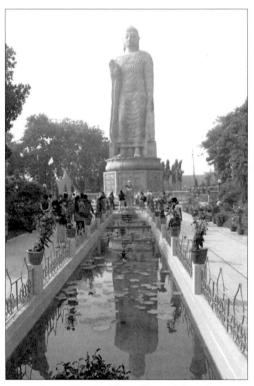

Statue of Lord Buddha, at Varanasi, Sarnath.

translators of their works and others, we owe an unconditional salute.

The same credit applies to T. W. Rhys Davids. Born in England in1843 as the eldest son of a Congregational clergyman from Wales, Rhys Davids studied Sanskrit under A. F. Stenzler, a distinguished scholar at the University of Bresla. As Professor of Pali at the University of London, and Founder of the Pali Text Society, Rhys Davids is credited as one of the first translators of early Buddhist texts.

The English word *mindfulness* was born in his hands. From the original Buddhist word *sati* was coined this giant of a word that, in the eyes of scores of scholars, has struggled to find the right home. Variously called or thought of as "possessing a good memory," "full of care," "heedful," "thoughtful," and "being conscious or aware," mindfulness was finally wrapped up in 2011 by *Oxford English Dictionary Online* as "the meditative state of being fully aware of the moment."

Smriti, the word that closely follows the heels of *sati*, is another example of various versions of an ill-understood word running amuck. From remembrance, reminiscence, and memory, this word, under the premises of the Sanskrit dictionary of Monier-Williams, is defined as "calling to mind" or "thinking of or upon."

Needless to say, to the Buddhist and any proponent of such eclectic terminologies, these are hardly comprehensive translations. As author Rupert Gethin wrote, "This is a matter of expedience in the absence of an exact English equivalent of Pali *sati* or Sanskrit *smriti*."

Caught amidst *sati* and *smriti*, mindfulness at its very subtlest falls in between a memory of the past and an attention to the present object of meditation in seamless continuity. In explicit terms, especially when it comes to its application, it can be likened to that of a "gatekeeper" that highlights qualities for what they are and to whom they belong.

I have warned you of the complexities of these worded thoughts traversing thousands of years under hundreds of upholders of its values. Lest we waddle in the mud of endless explanations for these

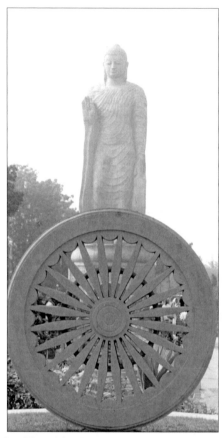

Lord Buddha and the Dharmachakra (Wheel of Law) at Sarnath.

words, we will retreat instead to the writings of Wangchuk Dorje, a Mahamudra teacher (1556–1601) as he put it in *Eliminating the Darkness of Ignorance* (*Ma rig mun sel*):

"Do not self-consciously try to accomplish anything, rather fix your mind like an eagle soaring. Be completely free from all expectations and worries. When you have no mental wandering, thoughts will not come. But when mental wandering occurs, then because your thoughts will come one after the other, try to recognize them for what they are as soon as they arise. In other words, stare right at them and then fix your mind as before. No matter what thoughts arise in this way, just recognize them for what they are. Place your attention right on them without thinking anything like, 'I must block them' or feeling happy or unhappy."[1]

Centuries down the road, Mahasi Sayadaw (1904–1982), a Burmese teacher affiliated with the tradition of modern Burmese insight meditation, gave to me what is one of the most visible displays of mindfulness meditation. He described mindfulness mediation as a journey where awareness progresses from the movement of the body to the movement of the mind.

"If you are thirsty while contemplating, notice the feeling, thirsty. When you intend to stand, intending. Keep the mind intently on the act of standing up, and mentally note, standing. When you look forward, after standing up straight, note looking, seeing. Should you intend to walk forward, intending. When you begin to step forward, mentally note each step as walking, walking, or left, right. It is important for you to be aware of every moment in each step from the beginning to the end when you walk. Adhere to the same procedure when strolling or when taking walking exercise. Try to make a mental note of each step in two sections as follows: lifting, putting, lifting, putting. When you have obtained sufficient practice in this manner of walking, then try to make a mental note of each step in three sections: lifting, pushing, or up, forward, down."[2]

---

1 *Berzin, 1978, p. 52*

2 Mahasi's *Practical insight meditation* (1971/1979, pp. 17–18) represents an English translation of instructions originally given and published in Burmese in 1944. The Burmese word translated as "noting" is *hmat*, which can mean "mark," "note," "keep in mind," "remember." (Gethin, R. Buddhist conceptualizations of mindfulness. In: RW Brown, JD Creswell, RM Ryan (eds.), *Handbook of mindfulness: Theory, research, and practice*. New York, NY: Guilford; 2014: 9–41.

The Experimental Evidence

As expected, increased awareness from mindfulness meditation was quickly captured in a joint experiment conducted in 2007 by the Institute of Neuroinformatics and Laboratory for Body and Mind, at Dalian University of Technology in China, and the Department of Psychology at the University of Oregon, in Eugene. Eighty healthy undergraduates at Dalian, without any training experience, participated in this study. They were randomly assigned to an experimental or control group (40:40). Forty experimental subjects continuously attended integrative body-mind training (IBMT), an ancient eastern contemplative tradition, involving body relaxation, mental imagery, and mindfulness training, for five days with 20 minutes of training per day. Forty control subjects were given the same number and length of group sessions, but received information from a compact disc about the relaxation of each body part.

A standardized computerized attention test measuring orienting, alerting, and the ability to resolve conflict (executive attention) was conducted before and after the experiment. The results were equivocal and to the point: the experimental group showed significantly greater improvement in executive attention and alertness after five days of IBMT than the relaxation control group. They also reported lower levels of anxiety, depression, anger, and fatigue, and high vigor when measured on the Profile of Mood States (POMS). Further, by measuring salivary cortisol levels and salivary immunoglobulin A levels (IgA), where IBMT participants showed significantly reduced levels, researchers logically inferred that stress levels were appreciably lower in the same group, compared to the control group.

But why select undergraduates? To my mind, this was a great scientific test. They wanted to obviate a possible bias that might creep in if the experiment involved senior citizens or devotees of mindfulness who were preconditioned to believe in the beneficial effects of meditation. A group of young men and women, devoid of these convictions and open to experimentation, was preferred and randomly selected.

The Mindfulness Meditator

At this juncture, let me delve a bit more deeply into the anatomical facets of the brain to take a firsthand look of what happens inside the mindfulness meditator. Our brain has two landmark areas called the Lateral Prefrontal Cortex (LPFC) and Parietal Cortex (PC). The Prefrontal Cortex (PFC), with its rich cortical and subcortical connections, performs numerous tasks, including the ability to initiate and carry out new and goal-directed patterns of behavior, sustained attention, and motor attention, among many others. The PFC's functions of encoding and retrieving memory appear as immensely significant. Intelligence as a complex construct comes out of PFC as well, along with regulating spontaneous speech, narrative expression, and verbal fluency.

This knowledge is of enormous relevance to us. Neuroimaging research has offered fascinating insights into the *attentional* effort of mindfulness meditators to engage various neural networks at various stages of practice. While the early stage of meditation involves both the LPFC and the PC, the advanced state of meditation completely shifts gears to turn its attention to the Anterior Cingulate Cortex (ACC) and the Ventral Striatum (VS), both of which fall under the "reward circuit" of our brain.

The ensured connections between these structures and the autonomic nervous system, along with their resulting ability to induce a parasympathetic dominance (the system that invokes a relaxation response), completes the circle of ecstasy.

The trip to heaven does not end here. Using diffusion tensor imaging to extensively map white matter tractography in the brain (an imaging method that uses the diffusion of water molecules to generate contrast in MRI images), several recent studies have shown that appropriate training actually resulted in changes in white matter efficiency and the integrity of the same caliber, as seen during child development. This breathtaking finding very simply stamps the judgment on the paper: Through its unparalleled ability to create white matter neuroplasticity, mindfulness meditation improves executive functioning and self-regulation.

Two words emerge graciously from *attention:* perception and memory. While the latter is the gold we are hunting for, the former carries equal importance.

What is perception?

Very simply, it refers to our ability to utilize our five senses to construct and perceive representations of the world in which we live.

Can you make the finest of the differences between two near-identical objects?

Or subjectively: *Can you perceive the finest of our overlapping emotions as individual entities?*

And then, the tempting question: *Can meditators exhibit better aptitudes of perception?*

Modern science would not bow down to any qualities without quantifying them. Scientist Katherine MacLean and her colleagues from the University of California jumped into the fray. Inspired by historical accounts of Buddhist contemplative tradition, the researchers focused on *Shamatha* practitioners who could stabilize their attention on a chosen stimulus, such as the tactile sensation of breathing, and subsequently enhance their perceived detail of that stimulus. In other words, they could "use introspection to monitor their quality of attention, recognize when attention has wandered, and guide attention back to the chosen stimulus."

What followed was a simulated experiment that was nothing short of a breakthrough.

Random individuals were chosen through online and newspaper advertisements. They belonged to all races and all ages. They were randomly allocated to two groups: one who underwent mindfulness meditation and the other who simply stood as controls. As they individually sat in a sound-attenuated, darkened testing room, a line—white, vertical, and centrally located—appeared on a screen with a dark background. This was followed soon after by a similar line, this time fractionally short.

While the longer line appeared frequently (hence called the non-target), the shorter "targeted" version came and went infrequently. The challenge was to detect the shorter line every time it appeared, randomly and callously, without any prior pattern. The task instructions emphasized the importance of speed and accuracy in responding to the short line by pressing the designated mouse button.

Participants received auditory feedback: a ding when they detected a target correctly and a whoosh when they missed a target or responded to a non-target. The researchers defined discrimination as the difference in visual angle between the threshold-level short line and the long line, with smaller threshold values representing a greater degree of discrimination.

The outcome?

Meditators showed far better discrimination qualities than the control group in persistently perceiving the shorter line when it appeared randomly on the screen. The experiment added to the overwhelming evidence that meditation training can improve aspects of attention, while also specifically suggesting the enhanced sustained-attention ability that has been linked to long-term meditation practice.

There is no escape now. We have systematically traversed the varied ranges of our mind based firmly on reproducible results. We need to close in—from attention to perception to the haunting target of memory. This time, scientists picked on U.S. Marines, specifically a cohort of pre-deployment military personnel. We shall meet them in a moment.

Explicit and Implicit Memory

Before we examine another study with all its intricacies, let us take a step back and dwell on the various shades of memory. Explicit memory or, more informally, declarative memory, is a tribute to our conscious recollection. Factual happenings or details, such as location, names, dates, telephone numbers, house address, social security numbers, and a multitude of other details, all fall under the umbrella of explicit memory.

I will not resist the temptation of reminding you that forgetting these factual details is nowhere near having Alzheimer's disease. God knows how many times anxious friends and senior citizens have asked me whether forgetting a telephone number is the first slender hint of onrushing Alzheimer's. I have strained my back and pained my throat to answer each time that Alzheimer's is a far more complex character than simple forgetfulness. Explicit memory regresses with time and age. It is a part of a physiological, almost graceful degeneration to which we *Homo sapiens* are subjected.

By contrast, implicit memory, also called emotional memory, is reluctant to leave our minds. How long do we remember *that* place because the most wonderful experience happened *there*? Chances are high you will recall such an incident, even if you are 90 years old and even if it happened in your youth when you were at the threshold of a world that was changing with every second. To the contrary, and on a darker note, I lose count of the number of people telling me how they fear flying, recalling the 9/11 tragedy. In short, emotional memories linger more than factual memories. And there is a science behind it.

Édouard Claparède and Henry Molaison:
Lives That Led the Way

Two stories stand out as classical representatives of these two types of memories and a primer of how the brain functions.

Édouard Claparède (1873–1940) was a Swiss neurologist, child psychologist, and educator who practiced medicine in Geneva, Switzerland. One of his female patients who suffered from amnesia secondary to brain damage challenged him relentlessly. She had all of her old memories as well as her basic reasoning skills, but she could not remember the recent past. Despite meeting the doctor on a regular basis, she had absolutely no recollection of the events—so much so that every time Dr. Claparède met her, he had to start all over again with an introduction to the rest of the formalities. Beyond the duration of the just-lived moment, the recent past was lost to her.

At this stage, Dr. Claparède thought of a novel experiment. He hid a pin in his palm when his patient arrived the next day. As he went through the ritualistic introductory motions that he repeated every day, he endeavored to shake hands with her. The moment the pin pricked his patient's palm, she withdrew her hand—an appropriate reaction. However, the following day was an absolute eye-opener for Dr. Claparède. His patient, as expected, and much to his frustration, did not remember the details of the previous day. However, most astonishingly—and gratifyingly—she refused to shake hands with him. While she failed to recollect any details of any past events, her subconscious feeling or memory of physical pain was intact.

Returning to our explanations of the two versions of memories, Dr. Claparède's patient had lost her explicit memory, but her implicit memory was intact!

This paved the road for one of the most talked-about research studies in the history of neuroscience, born out of a freak bicycle accident. If there is any example of surgical serendipity, this is it. It is also a tribute to our rigid frame of mind, where the human concerned is less known and less talked about, tucked behind a brain that became the center stage of one of the most dramatic behaviors and displays of intellect—and pride.

Famously known by his initials H. M., and hidden by the scientific world in an attempt to respect his privacy and the furious research born from the experiment, Henry Molaison was born a full-term baby, normal and healthy. His childhood was unremarkable and smooth until an accident at the age of nine put him in the throes of a transformation that was to be permanent yet intensely personal. He was playing outside his house one day when he was knocked down by a child riding a bicycle.

Henry fell on the ground and hit his head. He regained consciousness after five minutes, apparently normal, but not realizing that his life would change forever from that day. Henry started to seize soon after. Seizures that started off as the *petit mal* type, a French derivation of the phrase "little illness," where absence of seizures is accompanied by a sudden impairment of consciousness and a momentary cessation of ongoing activation. The seizures occurred regularly, without any respite, and with daily blackouts. The periodic but sudden interruption of his activities and the blank meaningless stares were typical of *petit mal* seizures. Medications seemed futile. In the years that followed, the episodes gravitated to full-blown, generalized, tonic clonic seizures.

Desperate and miserable, Henry's family doctor referred him to Dr. William Beecher Scoville, a neurosurgeon of repute based at the University of Hartford in Connecticut. Initially, Dr. Scoville fired all his guns and ordered all four medications to continue indefinitely: Dalantin, Phenobarbital, Tridione, and Mesantoin, all respected anti-epileptic medications in those days. However, nothing could harness the monstrous convulsions. Repeated EEG studies could not detect any foci of origin anywhere in the brain. In the meantime, despite the diurnal attacks, Henry graduated from high school and stepped into the outside world, desperate to taste normalcy. He briefly repaired electric motors and later worked on a typewriter assembly line. The seizures, fiercely resistant to all medications, continued hand in hand with his daily work, alternating from *petit mal* to intermittent generalized seizures.

The doctor decided it was time to enter Henry's brain. Henry, his family, and just about everyone who took care of him, agreed. The operation was considered experimental but inevitable, considering the irrepressible march of events tormenting Henry. Those were literally brain-bending times in the field of neuroscience. Wilder Penfield was then performing groundbreaking surgeries on epileptic and psychotic patients at the Montreal Neurological Institute. Dr. Scoville decided to go a step further. He planned to perform a bilateral resection of Henry's temporal lobes, unlike all previous one-sided brain surgeries.

Unfortunately, the tragedy of errors started right from here. The scalpel-wielding neurosurgeons had little knowledge of the functions of the hippocampus and amygdala, structures that were close to each other and routinely removed with a temporal lobectomy. On August 25, 1953, Dr. Scoville removed the following from Henry's brain:

+ the inner part of the temporal lobe,
+ most of the amygdaloid complex,
+ the hippocampal complex, except for two centimeters at the back,
+ the parahippocampal gyrus-entorhinal, perirhinal, and
+ the parahippocampal cortices, except for two centimeters at the back.

I include all these anatomical gory details simply because these very structures are considered the epicenters of various shades of human memory.

As history would soon reveal, Henry woke up, devoid of those mindless seizures yet trapped in a world of eternal forgetfulness. Medicine inadvertently struck gold through an intense personal tragedy.

What was unique in Henry's memory loss?

+ His short-term (immediate) memory was intact.
+ He failed to convert those short-term memories into long-term memories.
+ Post-surgery, he demonstrated a complete inability to form new memories.
+ His semantic memory prior to surgery was intact! (This refers to a portion of long-term memory that processes ideas and concepts not drawn from personal experience.)
+ His episodic memory prior to surgery showed deficits. (This refers to the recollection of biographical/autobiographical experiences and specific events.)
+ His spatial memory was deficient (the ability to remember the position or location of objects and places).
+ His performance on the Digit Span test (verbal working memory) was intact.
+ His IQ soared well above average.
+ His language, reasoning, and perceptual capacities were normal.

A panicked and thoroughly bemused Dr. Scoville reached out to Dr. Penfield in Canada, who sent one of his graduate students, neuropsychologist Dr. Brenda Milner of the Montreal Neurological Institute, to assess the situation. The meeting ignited a lifelong collaboration between the seeker and the sought, and in the ensuing 30 years, their work literally became a lighthouse in the stormy field of memory research.

Due to the fallibilities of his new brain, Henry had to be introduced to Brenda every day. They were cordial, affable, and interactive, but still needed formal pleasantries each day they met. On-the-spot procedural skills were perfect, but Henry soon forgot all that he learned. The trappings of his mind would not let him sustain any memory beyond 30 seconds. Henry floated between a retained remote past and a fickle-minded, uncertain present. Time seemed dulled to a long sleep. To Henry, Harry Truman would always be the President of the United States. His father's death shocked him repeatedly in renewed grief. Mirrors teased him, as he could not recognize the aging face that eventually looked back at him.

Henry's contribution to memory research was *immense*. By default or destiny, Henry had given his brain to save millions of minds. We will highlight some of the indispensable facts from this case:

+ Henry's deficient spatial memory established the importance of the hippocampus for spatial learning. Interestingly, when appropriately taught, he could accurately draw the map of the house where he lived, which meant that other the areas of the brain (parahippocampal gyrus, as established later) had taken over from his damaged hippocampus.
+ This meant that a healthy hippocampus was essential for vividly recollecting details.
+ Henry's intact procedural skills led to a deeper understanding that learning can take place without awareness (non-declarative memory).
+ His selectivity of remembering showed that the basic fractionation of short- and long-term memory are governed by a distinct and specialized memory circuit.

✦ From his unique dichotomies, we can comprehend the concept of semantic and episodic memory as distinctly different entities arising out of different anatomical substrates. Subsequent research has established that although the medial temporal lobe cradles the initial encoding, storage, and retrieval of both of these types of memories, subsequent consolidation places the semantic type in the cortex, while the episodic type continues to be dependent on its ancestral temporal lobe.

Henry had this identical fate. Clipped of his medial temporal lobes, he struggled with biographical and autobiographical details (episodic), while maintaining his general knowledge of the world (semantic).

Redefining "Attention"

Let us return to our Marines and witness the effects of mindfulness meditation on them.

In 2014, Dr. Amishi Jha from the Department of Psychology at the University of Miami, as well as Dr. Elizabeth Stanley from the Walsh School of Foreign Service and Department of Government at Georgetown University, conducted a seminal study on active-duty military service members preparing for combat. They looked at the effects of mindfulness training on what they called "attentional performance lapses" as subsequent to a task-unrelated thought. In simplistic terms, this is mind-wandering, despite being on duty.

While this might sound more like an oxymoron, we can appreciate the subtle yet consequential difference between standing at attention, a body posture that conveys motionless alertness, and a mind "at attention." In simplistic terms, after years of rigorous physical training, not all combatants would have the same unwavering resilience and concentration of the mind as is witnessed in physical terms.

These assume immeasurable importance and potentially carry tremendous risks when we appreciate that these vocations require extreme situational alertness. It is a daunting task to address low probability events and fast-changing circumstances.

Unfortunately, these mind-wandering episodes are not exotic incidents to be dismissed as an exception to the law. Experience-sampling studies have suggested that off-task thinking happens 30 percent to nearly 50 percent of our waking hours.

With that in mind, eighty healthy, active-duty U. S. marine male volunteers were recruited to participate in the Mindfulness-based Mind Fitness Training component of this project. The entire training and subsequent trials were conducted at Schofield Barracks in Hawaii, between eight to ten months prior to the participants' deployment to Afghanistan.

While one group received an eight-hour, eight-week variant of the mindfulness-based mind fitness training, the second group received training that was essentially didactic, emphasizing stress management and resilience. The third group acted as a control, with none of the prior interventions offered.

A Sustained Attention to Response Task (SART) performance was assigned to all participants. The results unequivocally showed that compared to the no-training control group, the military cohorts who received mindfulness training had significantly fewer performance lapses. Results were equally positive for those in the training-focused "Mindfulness Training," who performed significantly better than those who only received the didactic course.

Clinical Applications on Alzheimer's

How does any of this help in my grandma's impending dementia?

Mindfulness meditation helps the failing mind in two primary ways. Alterations in brain nerve cells (neuroplasticity) and the brain waves caused by meditation offer a direct benefit in terms of better concentration, focus, and memory. Mindfulness meditation also has a secondary effect because it decreases the risk factors that accelerate Alzheimer's disease. High blood pressure, high cholesterol, high cortisol levels, stress, and obesity have all been implicated in the establishment of full-blown Alzheimer's.

In a society where salt (sodium) is sprinkled on virtually every food we eat in fairly large doses, where stress has become a way of life, high blood pressure is a natural result. Intense interaction and collaboration between genes, environment, lifestyle, and eating habits have brought hyperlipidemia and diabetes to the forefront. Not surprisingly, medications to combat these illnesses have poured out of pharmaceutical companies with a vengeance. They have been lifesaving, not just in bringing down the numbers, but more importantly, in thwarting the complications that arise out of it, be they coronary or vascular. Yet, true to the colors of a chemical compound, they also offer side effects, drug interactions, and "tolerance issues."

Can meditation be used as a complementary measure?

Can it prevent or minimize our dependence on drugs?

Strong evidence of its anti-hypertensive benefits was found in research conducted at Kent State University in Ohio. Published in the 2013 October issue of *Psychosomatic Medicine: Journal of Biobehavioral Medicine*, the study showed that mindfulness meditation, along with yoga techniques, lowered the blood pressure on patients suffering from pre-hypertension, a state defined as blood pressure that is higher than normal but not high enough to require drug therapy. Pre-hypertension is associated not only with Alzheimer's, but with a wide range of heart disease and other cardiovascular problems.

The "active" group of patients undertook eight group sessions comprised of body scan exercises, sitting meditation, and yoga exercises for two-and-a-half hours per week. They were also encouraged to perform mindfulness exercises at home. The "comparison" group received lifestyle advice plus a muscle-relaxation activity. The results showed that patients in the mindfulness-based intervention group had significant reductions in clinic-based blood pressure measurements.

Equally encouraging were the effects of Raja yoga meditation (a form of mindfulness meditation) on cholesterol, another risk factor for Alzheimer's disease. In a study conducted at B. J. Medical College and Civil Hospital in India, 49 female patients were divided into non-meditators (those who had never done any kind of meditation), short-term meditators (meditating for six months to five years), and long-term meditators (meditating for more than five years). The results indicated that both serum cholesterol and low-density lipoprotein-cholesterol were significantly lowered in both short- and long-term meditators, as compared to non-meditators, especially in post-menopausal women.

As a precursor to Alzheimer's, stroke, coronary artery diseases, diabetes, and high blood pressure, obesity has truly been the scourge of our society. While anti-obesity pills, weight-reducing surgery, and nutritional supplements have taken center stage, meditation has emerged as a strong, risk-free option for reducing body weight.

A pioneering research trial, performed at both the University of California and Indiana State University, tested the effects of mindfulness meditation on belly fat among overweight and obese women. The intervention program consisted of nine, two-and-a-half-hour classes and one seven-hour silent day of guided meditation practice. Participants were also led through guided meditations as a way to introduce mindful eating practices, such as paying attention to the physical sensations of hunger, stomach fullness, taste satisfaction, and food cravings.

The results showed that intervention participants who reported the greatest improvements in mindfulness meditation had the largest reductions in abdominal fat. This clearly supported the strength of mind over matter. Furthermore, significant reductions in a body hormone related to stress were noted, leading to reductions in abdominal fat.

Stress, as we will see in more detail later, is virtually the epicenter of an ever-brewing storm. This risk factor can be singled out as relentless, ruthless, and unstoppable. Whether it occurs as a generalized anxiety disorder or as a consequence of trauma, stress has an obvious psychological connotation to it. However, stress has impacts well beyond the psychiatric realm. It can push the mind into dementia.

According to Dr. Elizabeth Hoge, a psychiatrist at the Center for Anxiety and Traumatic Stress Disorders at Massachusetts General Hospital, and an assistant professor of psychiatry at Harvard Medical School, "People with anxiety have a problem dealing with distracting thoughts that have too much power. . . . They can't distinguish between a problem-solving thought and a nagging worry that has no benefit."

Dr. Hoge indicated that if one has unproductive worries, one can self-train to experience those thoughts in a completely different way, as she explains:

"You might think 'I'm late, I might lose my job if I don't get there on time, and it will be a disaster!' Mindfulness teaches you to recognize, 'Oh, there's that thought again. I've been here before. But it's just that—a thought, and not a part of my core self.'"

The effects of meditation on reducing stress have been conclusively proven in multiple trials. In one of the most extensive meta-analyses ever conducted, researchers from Johns Hopkins University sifted through nearly 19,000 meditation studies and 47 trials that met the criteria for well-designed studies. Published in the March 2014 issue of the *Journal of American Medical Association (JAMA)*, the findings clearly showed that mindfulness meditation eases spsychological stresses, such as anxiety, depression, and pain.

Further studies have examined participants with generalized anxiety disorder, a condition marked by persistent worries, insomnia, and irritability. Those who entered a mindfulness-based stress-reduction program had significant reductions in their anxiety symptoms. By contrast, people who were taught general stress-management techniques did not experience similar reductions.

Inspired By the Himalayas

As we have witnessed already, by far the most rewarding research into mindfulness meditation examines its capability to rewire structure and functions of the brain. If you endeavor to track the genesis of all these studies, you would probably find yourself at the foot of the Himalayas. There resides, amid the encircling embrace of the sublime snowy ranges, the Fourteenth Dalai Lama, leader of Tibetan Buddhism.

In 2005, the Dalai Lama was invited to the annual meeting of the Society for Neuroscience in Washington, D. C. In the speech he delivered on that breezy November evening, he raised two pressing topics.

The first involved a set of pivotal questions.

"What relation could there be between Buddhism, an ancient Indian philosophical and spiritual tradition, and modern science?

What possible benefit could there be for a scientific discipline, such as neuroscience, in engaging in dialogue with Buddhist contemplative tradition?"

Second was his fervent plea to the scientific world:

"It is all too evident that our moral thinking simply has not been able to keep pace with such rapid progress in our acquisition of knowledge and power. Yet the ramifications of these new findings and their applications are so far-reaching that they relate to the very conception of human nature and the preservation of the human species. We must find a way of bringing fundamental humanitarian and ethical considerations to bear upon the direction of scientific development, especially in the life sciences."

The Dalai Lama was voicing the concerns of many scholars who struggle with the ethical aspects of scientific advances.

How honest are we in our scientific pursuits?

What forms the nucleus of such explorations—service to humanity or acquisition of power?

Fanaticism, be it religious or scientific, has forever troubled the world. The peaks and pinnacles of glorious discoveries have not been able to cure the mud and mire of our greed and bigotry.

Can spirituality help science?

This glorious son of Buddha chose to take the battle head on. Like an apostle, the Dalai Lama sent his own soldiers, Tibetan Buddhist monks, to Richard Davidson's Waisman Laboratory for Brain Imaging and Behavior in Wisconsin.

Let's examine what the researchers found. They used functional magnetic resonance imaging (fMRI) requiring a high field-strength MRI scanner equipped with appropriate pulse sequences. This equipment, which acquires data rapidly, was used to assess and measure changes. Further, they measured brain electrical activity, using a high-density recording system with between 64 and 256 electrodes on the scalp surface.

The results were not just overwhelming. To the scientists, it must have felt like they were discovering life on another planet. Research from this unusual sample suggested that, over the course of meditating for tens of thousands of hours, long-term practitioners actually altered the structure and function of their brains. The results clearly demonstrated activation in specific multiple brain regions involved in monitoring, engaging attention, and attentional orienting.

The reports must have shaken the scientific fraternity. Studies and trials poured in from all corners of the globe.

In 2010, related research studies were conducted at the Institute of Psychiatry at the University of Bologna in Italy. They showed that the early phases of mindfulness training, when a person is learning how to focus his attention, are associated with significant improvements in focused attention. In addition, the mature phases of mindfulness training are associated with improved, sustained attention. The tests also showed that mindfulness meditation practices can enhance a person's working memory capacity, thereby enhancing the ability to execute the functions of daily living.

In 2013, further studies from Beth Israel Deaconess Medical Center's Cognitive Neurology Unit in Boston, Massachusetts, revealed that, compared to a control group, Mindfulness-Based Stress Reduction, a combination of mindfulness meditation, body awareness, and yoga, resulted in increased gray matter in the left hippocampus, a brain area strongly involved in learning and memory.

Three years later, research from the Department of Psychiatry and Psychotherapy at the University of Margburg in Germany pointed to enhancement of those areas of the brain responsible for the process of mindfulness. Using Diffusion Tensor Imaging (a diagnostic tool used to characterize microstructural changes or differences in neuropathology), meditators, as opposed to non-meditators, showed increased white matter connectivity in those key regions of the brain involved in mindfulness, such as the thalamus, insula, amygdala, hippocampus, and anterior cingulate cortex.

From all these institutional findings emerges one gracious fact we all need to know. Those areas of the brain that play significant roles in harnessing concentration, attention, and focusing are the ones that receive the most comprehensive benefit from meditation. To prevent the brain sinking into dementia, meditation is the path to walk.

Transcendental Meditation

In terms of how Transcendental Meditation (TM) arrests the development of Alzheimer's, we need to remind ourselves of two parallel events that accompany the disease.

First, Alzheimer's is not just about its sufferers forgetting things. An entire spectrum of emotions descend on those disturbed minds. Afflicted patients can harbor agitation, personality changes, severe depression, stress, an inability to execute complex functions, and many other cognitive deficiencies. Each of these components serves to escalate the other.

Second, Alzheimer's is not a solitary disease. The whole family suffers with it. The caregiver in particular—in most cases, spouses or children—suffer these pangs with equal intensity. They are at the receiving end of the disease as much as their loved one.

TM endeavors to approach and address both of these groups. Equally relevant is the reminder that Alzheimer's, in its early stage, which we know as mild cognitive impairment (MCI), may not even be considered dementia. The subtle effects, involving either emotions or intellect or personalities, come into consideration years before the complete dementia gels.

Transcendental meditation has enjoyed much publicity. In contrast to mindfulness meditation, in which distracting thoughts and feelings are not ignored but are acknowledged and observed nonjudgmentally, TM has a far simpler approach. Based on ancient Indian traditions, it was developed by Maharishi Mahesh Yogi in the second half of the twentieth century.

It essentially entails the repetition of a *mantra* for 15 to 20 minutes, twice a day, with the eyes closed. Mantras are sounds or simple sentences that help the meditating person stay focused. Attention is paid to overcoming our constant outpouring of thoughts and to discover their source, which is felt as a moment of pure conscious-ness, absolutely free of any content.

Simplicity and effortlessness emerge as hallmarks of this type of meditation. If we go back to a mind affected by mild cognitive impair-ment, we would appreciate that the undemanding approaches of TM that do not lean on an intact and superior intellect would be ideal ref-uges to adopt. In fact, the ideologies of TM endorse rather than resist the natural proclivity of the human mind to drift toward happiness.

The idea is that the wandering mind will find its way to happi-ness, drawn by the "increasing charm" of its own blissful depths. The journey is a slow, smooth transition, from pure consciousness to a zone where one's awareness is suspended. With further practice, a permeation follows, allowing entrance into a space that is uncircum-scribed and limitless, free from the shackles of thoughts, images, or sensory objects.

For decades, the easy-to-learn repetition of a few words during meditation sessions has captivated followers around the globe. The most famous were the Beatles. For all four—Paul McCartney, John Lennon, George Harrison, and Ringo Starr—their time spent in TM helped create moments of peace amid the vicious cycle of frenzied mobs, drugs, and depression.

In an interview with host David Frost on a BBC show in 1968, both Lennon and Harrison talked of an elevated "energy" that became their instant companions once they learned the techniques of TM.

Frost asked, "There were two things Maharishi said this morn-ing that were the result of people meditating, following his system of meditation. The two things he claimed were serenity and energy. Have you found them?"

Lennon replied: "The energy that I've found doing meditation, you know, has been there before—only that I could access it only during good days when everything was going well. With meditation,

I find that it could well be pouring down rain, and it is still the same amount."

Harrison had a similar answer: "The energy is latently there every day, anyway. So meditation is just a natural process of contacting it. By doing it each day, you give yourself a chance of contacting this energy and giving it to yourself a little more. Consequently you're able to do whatever you normally do—just with a little bit more happiness, maybe."

For McCartney, the effects were more profound and lasting. In an interview with director David Lynch, McCartney, who still practices meditation every day, swore by its effects: "I think it's always very good to get a sort of still moment in your day. Whenever I have a chance in a busy schedule, I'll do it, if I'm not rushing out the door with some crazy stuff to do. But yeah, I always like to take a moment and just meditate. Transcendental Meditation is a good thing."

Following the lead of the Beatles, TM invaded all walks of our society, from business executives to teachers to students of all kinds. As one can surmise easily, the rapidity of its global influence hinges on a technique that is easily grasped and user-friendly.

Therapeutically, *transcendental* matches *mindfulness* trial by trial. Interesting results have come from the Division of Endocrinology and Molecular Medicine of the College of Medicine at the University of Kentucky. In 2007, a research study team, led by primary investigator, Dr. J. W. Anderson, revealed that the regular practice of TM strongly reduces blood pressure.

Almost simultaneously, compelling results emerged from the Center for Natural Medicine and Prevention at Maharishi University of Management in Fairfield, Iowa, showing decreased levels of cholesterol following TM practice.

Three years later, a study by the University of Pennsylvania Medical Center demonstrated significant cerebral blood flow differences between long-term meditators and non-meditators. Identical to what was seen in research involving mindfulness mediation, here too with TM, scientists observed changes in long-term meditators in structures that underlay the attention network, as well as those relating to autonomic function, such as the heart rate, digestion, and respiratory rate, among others, as well as emotion.

A Coping Tool

To my eighty-year-old patient, Ronald Ricardo, it boiled down to "just feeling goddarn good." Ronald had had his share of health issues, including diabetes, hypertension, and high cholesterol. They were all under control because he regularly took his medications, but Ronald was unusually reticent during one of his visits to my office.

"Is everything okay with you, Mr. Ricardo?"

No answer. Only a nod.

The physical examination was unremarkable except a heart rate that sped well over 100 beats per minute.

"You seem to be tense. Your heart is racing away."

"I guess I am," he whispered.

"What's bothering you, Ronald?"

"Nothing specific, Doctor. My belly hurts, my chest hurts. I am forgetting things like crazy. I am a mess. . . ."

The last sentence was whispered with an exasperated undertone.

The story that came out was typical. His family-run restaurant had been on a steep downward slope. His grandson was on drugs. He had recently lost his sister, with whom he was very close. He was constantly forgetting where he kept his glasses and notebook. In short, he was stressed out.

Before I could address his plethora of ailments, he blurted out, "But the last thing I want you to prescribe is Xanax!"

I wasn't surprised by his answer, as I knew that Mr. Ricardo would be the last person to take refuge in drugs.

"What are your thoughts on meditation?" I asked him softly.

"Way too complicated for me," came his terse reply.

"What if it's way too simplistic by your standards?" I said.

Suddenly, he smiled. What a relief, I thought, as he cleared his throat.

"What's on your mind, Doc? Time for you to talk."

I explained the benefits of Transcendental Meditation as a risk-free practice that was so simple to do Mr. Ricardo agreed to a trial run and I provided him with the details of a nearby center.

In the past three years, remarkable changes have happened in Ronald's life, despite the fact that his family restaurant is still struggling and his grandson is still fighting to be clean.

"I am so much at peace," he told me during his last visit. "I feel so unstressed."

This is exactly why Transcendental Meditation is emerging as a popular therapy to address the perils of a stressful life. Even short trials have generated positive effects. A mere eight-week meditation training study at Massachusetts General Hospital showed a significant decrease in activation in the right amygdala (a part of the brain important for emotions), supporting the hypothesis that meditation can improve emotional stability and response to stress.

As Dr. Fred Davis, a leading neurologist and author of the book *Your Brain Is a River, Not a Rock*, commented, "What I think Transcendental Meditation is doing is erasing that line between challenge and stress. You can take on increasingly more and more challenge without it becoming stressful. I think some of that is because you never have the perception that it's too much; you never have the perception that this experience is going to overtake you."

Clint Eastwood, film actor and disciple of TM, had the same thoughts: "I've been using it for almost 40 years now and I think it's a great tool for anyone to have, to be able to *utilize as a tool for stress.* Stress, of course, comes with almost every business."

The dance and dominance of meditation could not have been timelier. Studies coming out of the Department of Biostatistics at Johns Hopkins Bloomberg School of Public Health revealed that delaying the onset of Alzheimer's disease by only a year would yield nine million fewer cases by 2050. They also stated something more profound: that the prevention of dementia may be more effective with TM than with current drug treatments.

Answers Still on the Horizon

We have flooded ourselves with facts and figures, straining to prove how meditation shines under the microscope. Yet we know that objective results can take the pursuit of truth only so far. We also know that over and above these facts and figures are areas, uncharted but evolving, beyond the laboratory but within the premises of a seeking mind, that hinge on a willingness to trespass. For the sake of truth, we experiment, yet a greater truth eludes the experimental mind.

My first meeting with Dr. Walter Jackson Freeman III took place in October 1999, under a cloudy Brooklyn sky on the premises of Long Island University. He was a semi-retired theoretical neuroscientist, biologist, and philosopher who worked in the labs of the University of California at Berkeley, pioneering research in how brains generate meaning. I was humbled by his aura of wisdom that instantly and happily humbled this onlooker. He smiled away most of my audacious inquiries as if they were bottles of moonlight. The ones that he chose to respond to were pure honey.

Later, as we ambled away from campus and settled down in a nearby Thai restaurant, we discussed his work. Among all his legendary works on chaotic dynamics, his writings on the fundamental aspects of happiness had pounced on me like one bright kid—attractive, willing, and decidedly daring. Misquoted, misjudged, misunderstood, and misled, the hunger for happiness has been the source of endless misery. Our conversations drifted to mind and memory, and this time it was his turn to plunge in with the typical childlike eagerness of a visionary.

Dr. Freeman talked about his landmark article, "Consciousness, intentionality, and causality." In it, he had defined consciousness as "a global internal state variable composed of a sequence of momentary states of awareness."

What is a "global state variable"?

According to Dr. Freeman, this involves "sensations, images, feelings, thoughts and beliefs," that "constitute the experience of causation."

"Do these make sense to you?" he asked me good-humoredly.

Of course it did. In fact, I was happily surprised at how close it came to the definitions and viewpoints of what had been felt and preached in the ancient past. Consciousness, or what is called *citta* in Sanskrit, has being viewed as having the potential to know and think. *Citta* has no matter, no tangible form, or any place in which to remain. It is continuously changing, and travels unendingly without beginning or end.

To switch back to Dr. Freeman's views, the brain evolves in a back-and-forth process of our reacting to sensations and images with feelings, thoughts, and beliefs. Call it consciousness, soul, or spirit—the attributes pertaining to the mind depend on one's *own* journey.

This conclusion takes on tremendous importance when considering the art of meditation. Unlike a pharmaceutical drug that is swallowed with little personal initiative, meditation is an individual process that requires one's *own* motivation and commitment. *You* are challenging *your* mind, thus repairing it.

An event of paramount significance emerged from these concepts.

Freeman had often quoted British mathematician Sir Roger Penrose, who in his 1994 book titled *The Emperor's New Mind* argued that known laws of physics are inadequate to explain the phenomenon of consciousness. He based this on claims that consciousness transcends formal logic. He took refuge in the principles of quantum theory as an alternative process through which consciousness could arise.

In a grand coincidence, thousands of miles away across the Atlantic Ocean, anesthesiologist and University of Arizona professor Stuart Hameroff was investing all his intellectual and creative energies on the essences of microtubules—subneuronal and vital cytoskeleton components that he believed could be the cradle of our information processing system. He reasoned that the mystery of consciousness might lie in understanding these microtubules in brain cells, functioning at both the molecular and supramolecular levels.

The two were destined to meet, and did so in 1992. What followed was at once magical. Hameroff lent his microtubules to Penrose's quantum theory, giving birth to the Orchestrated Objective Reduction (Orch-OR) model of consciousness. For the next two years, they researched the premise that consciousness is the result of the presence of quantum vibrations in infinitely small structures of the central nervous system, called *microtubules*. At a fundamental level, this meant that consciousness was derived from deeper-level, finer-scaled quantum activities inside cells, most prevalent in the neurons.

In undeterred audacity, they dumped mainstream ideas to demonstrate that consciousness was based on non-computable quantum processing—and hence cannot be reproduced by computer logic—performed by qubits (a unit of quantum information), formed collectively on cellular microtubules, a process significantly amplified in the neurons. While critics instantly sharpened their knives, calling the theory short-sighted and lacking in credibility, physicist Dr. Anirban Bandyopadhyay, working in his laboratory in the National Institute of Material Sciences in Tsukuba, Japan (and now at MIT), jumped to their rescue, corroborating the pair's theory with the added suggestions that even electroencephalogram (EEG) rhythms were derived from deeper-level microtubule vibrations. More work came from the laboratory of Roderick G. Eckenhoff, M.D., at the University of Pennsylvania. Research there showed that anesthesia, which selectively erases consciousness while sparing non-conscious brain activities, also acts via microtubules in brain neurons. These were enough for trigger-happy scientists to cut loose. Close to these near-revolutionary theories came clinical trials of brief brain stimulation aimed at microtubule resonances using transcranial ultrasound.

"Did consciousness evolve from complex computations among brain neurons, as most scientists assert?" a euphoric Hameroff and Penrose asked the world, "or has consciousness, in some sense, been here all along, as spiritual approaches maintain?"

Science had suddenly stumbled into the backyard of a beyond that is also infinitely close. In an instant, microtubules smelled like the grass where Buddha and his consciousness once sat, and all this became infinitely relevant to sufferers of Alzheimer's. The terrifying spectacles of amyloid plaques wrecking these very microtubules confronted us in an unblinking stare.

Powerful, mind-bending questions emerged.

Can meditation, with its potential for neuroplasticity (alterations of nerve cells), replenish the dwindling quantum energy of the microtubules plagued by the onset of Alzheimer's?

Can meditation prevent *degeneration, with its boundless capability to crystallize energy, before Alzheimer's arrives?*

Can meditative electrical waves be preserved in the microtubules?

The possibilities are endless, and going by the outpourings of positive research, we have every reason to be hopeful.

We have seen this process before. Ancient sages advocated practices that rigorous scientific study later found immeasurably beneficial. Siddhartha lived in an age when nerve endings, let alone microtubules, were unknown. Yet the calm and increased focus of sitting alone and concentrating for long periods produced results that performed better than any laboratory-produced compound.

It is time to prescribe meditation.

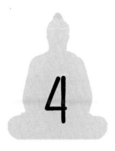

FROM NALANDA TO HARVARD UNIVERSITY: YOGA'S BREATHTAKING JOURNEY

Yoga is the cessation of the movements of the mind.
Then there is abiding in the Seer's own form.

—Patañjali, The Yoga Sutras of Patanjali

About fifty-five miles southeast of Patna, the present capital city of the state of Bihar in India, lies Rajgir, a town surrounded by silent mountains and undulating greens. This is where Nalanda University was born in the fifth century BC, one of the earliest scholarly homes of human civilization. Under the patronage of the kings of the Gupta Dynasty, fashionably called the Golden Era of Indian History, and buoyed by the sacred teachings of Lord Buddha, knowledge, bloomed like a rich harvest spanning centuries to follow.

At Nalanda University, the gathering of wisdom was a guiding force, embracing both the mind and the spirit. It attracted and

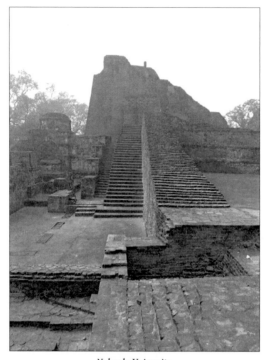

Nalanda University.

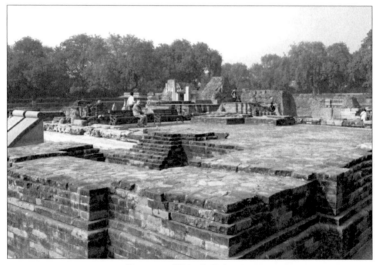

Remnants of Nalanda University.

provoked the finest of minds. Philosophy, music, spirituality, mathematics, astronomy, logic—all possible branches of knowledge—were assembled in eight separate compounds and ten temples, along with many other meditation halls and classrooms. In a majestic display of architectural brilliance, lofty, red brick walls surrounded a yawning campus that harbored lakes and ponds amid monasteries and classrooms, where students studied and lived. Scholars came from diverse parts of the world, such as China, Tibet, Persia, and Greece, to be happily trapped in an endless academic trance.

In its heyday, this residential university harbored 10,000 students and 2,000 teachers, among them the Lord Buddha. As might be imagined, most outstanding of all was the university library, a structural masterpiece divided into three buildings with exclusive sections for Hindu and Buddhist scholars.

The Beginnings of Yoga

Yoga flourished in this repository of boundless knowledge. Through the dreamy eyes of passing centuries and fables, history may not provide all the concrete facts of this way of life that has recently found a meaningful existence in modern civilization. Yet, its fundamental truths have stood the test of time.

As the father or founder of yoga, the Indian sage Patanjali compiled 195 *sutras*, which serve as a framework for integrating yoga into the daily routine of an ethical life. The exact date of the compilation of the yoga *sutras* is not known. However, it is believed they were written around 200 BC.

The core of Patanjali's teachings lies in the eight-fold path of yoga. Called the eight limbs of *Ashtang Yoga*, these comprise various shades of life that are to be achieved sequentially to pursue a meaningful and purposeful life. Encompassing *yamas* (ethical disciplines), *niyamas* (individual observances), *asanas* (postures), *pranayama* (breath control), *pratyahara* (withdrawal of senses), *dharana* (concentration), and *dhyana* (meditation), the eighth limb is *samadhi*, the final bow from life leading to self-realization or enlightenment.

All these could be easily passed off as spiritual offerings typical of an era with much exalted imagination and little scientific underpinnings. But because this somewhat folkloric figure Patanjali was also a physician, we are enticed to probe more deeply into his writings. The fact that his proposed eight limbs of knowledge were meant to be a prescription for both physical and moral health goads us to seek more.

Justifiably, under the scrutinizing eyes of Western scientific literature, yoga as a concept became trimmed into a set of values comprised of breathing techniques, postures, strengthening exercises, and meditation. It was trimmed not because the West had a problem with the East, but because all those techniques and postures were scientifically found to be beneficial to humankind. This has elevated yoga to a level of profound pragmatism, free from the intrusions of religious scruples and bickering.

The most common forms of yoga practiced in the West are the physical postures and breathing practices of what is called *Hatha Yoga*. Being more physical than the other forms, Hatha Yoga focuses on the conscious prolongation of inhalation, breath retention, and exhalation. The physicality of yoga, as depicted through *asanas* or postures, rests on the concept of stretching and strengthening different parts of the body, thereby inviting a surplus of oxygenated blood to the organs, thereby rejuvenating the nervous system. The abdominal breathing technique and focus of awareness to the present physical experience form the mental counterparts.

This present-focused sensory awareness resonates with the Buddhist philosophy of mindfulness meditation. This is a happy meeting place that should not surprise us, knowing what Nalanda University originally sought and served.

Yoga's Tryst
with Harvard University

But how did yoga make its way to the West? The answer lies at the foundation of Western acceptance. Most fittingly, the honors fell on a modern-day Indian monk who was also one of the greatest scientific minds the country has produced. Fashionably called Vivekananda by the West, this exquisitely gifted soul captivated intellectual and spiritual Americans with his charming eloquence and bold convictions.

On August 25, 1893, Vivekananda met John Henry Wright, who wore America's finest scholarly hat of his time as Dean of Graduate Arts and Sciences at Harvard University. Their brief encounter left Professor Wright amazed by Vivekananda's profound knowledge and he urged him to speak at the upcoming Parliament of the World's Religions Summit in Chicago.

What followed was a complete fairytale, albeit very *American*. When Vivekananda told Wright that he did not have any bona fide credentials to attend the Parliament, Wright reportedly told him: "To ask you, Swami, for your credentials is like asking the sun about its right to shine." Then Wright himself wrote a letter of introduction to the chairman of the Parliament and suggested that he invite Vivekananda as a speaker, describing him as "more learned than all our learned professors put together."

Vivekananda's appearance laid the foundation of a bridge that became the gateway for oriental philosophy's advent in the West. Not surprisingly, both Harvard and Columbia University offered Vivekananda the Chairmanship of Eastern Philosophy at their respective institutions—positions that were politely declined.

Yet the seed Vivekananda had sown was destined to bloom. As we will soon see, Harvard University emerged as the virtual epicenter of health management through its mind-body concept, as inspired by Vivekananda. Of his many teachings, his discourses on Raja Yoga—roughly translated as "Union by mental mastery"—has stood the test of time. As Vivekananda indicates, it is the method of mental concentration involving the power to bring the consciousness under submission through the practice of the eight steps that Patanjali described in his yoga *sutras*. Of these, the one he stressed the most was *Pranayama*, or breath control.

Pranayama forms the pivot of yoga's triumphant strides into the modern practice of medicine. Composed from two Sanskrit words—*prana*. meaning life force (noted particularly as the breath), and either *yama* (to restrain or control the *prana*, implying a set of breathing techniques where the breath is intentionally altered to produce specific results), or the negative form, *ayāma* (to extend or draw out, as in extension of the life force), *Pranayama* has eased its way into every major university health center today.

Treasures from Nalanda University

In his research on the journey of meditation, Joseph Loizzo, from the Center of Integrative Medicine at Weill Cornell Medical College, traces this exact path from the premises of Nalanda University to the present-day marriage of conventional research and contemplative tradition. He explores the Nalanda tradition that was born in India and is now preserved in Tibet, precisely because its naturalistic theories and empirical methods best bridge the chasm between an objective science and a subjective contemplation.

According to Dr. Loizzo, the beauty of the Nalanda type of

contemplative tradition lies "in the less theistic explanatory language, and a more extensive and continuous academic tradition of oral and written commentary."

The Avon Foundation recently funded a Weil Cornell Center pilot study on 68 breast cancer survivors. Predictably, they suffered from stress, depression, and anxiety—all justifiable manifestations of the wild whirl of continued affliction. Researchers found that, compared to any other psychosocial intervention studies, including mindfulness-based stress reductions, aerobic exercises, and traditional antidepressants, the Nalanda Program produced stronger effects on quality of life and traumatic avoidances.

What exactly did the Nalanda Program entail? Before we answer and delineate the details, we must consider an alternate viewpoint.

Not long ago, neuroscience looked upon any response to a stressful situation as a recurring event secondary to two events. One comprised a range of "learned concepts" reflecting an individual's view of self and the surrounding society that included age, gender, ethnicity, self-involvement, self-efficacy, socioeconomic status, and social support. The second involved the sufferer's reaction to the suffering, including anxiety, hostility, shame, helplessness, hopelessness, or depression, and his or her coping mechanisms. These, according to conventional beliefs, fashioned the mind into an adaptive framework, like the long-term conditioning of one's own cognition, affect, and behaviors to dictate stereotypical habits of stress reactivity.

Current cognitive behavioral models have changed, not that they have adopted anything new or jazzy. Rather, they have arched thousands of years back to what prevailed on the premises of Nalanda University. In contrast to the perfunctory assumption that all disease states, including stress, are external elements that provoke an outward reaction, this Indo-Tibetan tradition sees them as internal dysregulations coming out of a failure to adapt. They are endemic situations that are inherent and unique in an individual when exacerbated by illness, aging, and dying.

This *was* the vintage medicine of the past—this quiet acknowledgment that suffering, aging, and death are existential human conditions and not "alien intrusions" to be damaged, denied, or dented. Modern medicine suffers from a proletariat attitude, where all humans, all diseases, and all treatments are standardized and set in stone. The singular sensitiveness of a soul is completely ignored.

All too often, this tunnel vision prompts resistance to treatment.

The Components of Individualism and Adaptation

So, what are the thoughts of the Indo-Tibetan science of stress healing? If you keep in mind the two cushioning points of traditional medicine, namely individualism and adaptation, the thoughts will flow in pleasing reveries. Contrasting them with the now defunct reactionary concept of stress, they will look something like this:

Reactionary	Adaptation
Self-Involvement	Self-Knowledge
Senseless Illness	Meaningful Illness
Mindless Reproduction	Mindful Generation
Compulsive Life	Liberated Life
Obsessive Clinging	Voluntary Release
Addictive Craving	Sober Renunciation
Negative Emotion	Positive Emotion
Alienated Consciousness	Connected Consciousness
Isolated Self-Construct	Relaxed Self-Construct
Distorted Perception	Realistic Perception
Reactive Sensation	Proactive Sensation

These changing concepts offered a commanding footing for concerted action. Accordingly, Dr. Joseph Laizzo and his team taught cancer survivors a series of eight skills or techniques and twelve insights or strategies in a twenty-week contemplative learning program. Researchers broke the program up into two modules, which included eight weekly group classes focusing on teaching meditative techniques and an additional twelve weekly classes dedicated to lectures, discussions, and experiential learning exercises, with weekly homework consisting of daily practice through guided meditation.

Dr. Lazzio's intention was clear, objective, and reflective of the unique Tibetan style of thought. Individuals were taught insights and skills that were suited to their *own* daily needs and challenges.

The fundamental ingredients of these techniques included developing skills of heightened attention, deep breathing, and visualization-based contemplative learning. This integrative approach improved not only overall well-being, but also the emotional and functional well-being of the individuals, as measured by standard scales used to assess quality of life in cancer patients.

To me, something more concrete and deep emerges from these implications. The results also suggest that the whole theology of Indo-Tibetan mind-body practices could be successfully absorbed by contemporary Westerners to be implemented in their overall quality of life. It is this very accessibility to these techniques that makes yoga so universally and easily adoptable.

Stress: The Inescapable Scourge

Why are we always so stressed out?

Almost like a legacy, some diseases proclaim, proliferate, and prevail eternally. Heart attack, stroke, cancer—the list is growing. These are the powerhouses of the medical world that dictate terms. They motivate huge interests, research papers, and industries. But beneath these established dynasties flourish smaller families, existing between raindrops, unassuming, almost sly—the quintessential king-breakers, as we say.

In our medical fraternity, we call them "risk factors." Stress, among all these, hogs the limelight. It has an identity of its own. Undefined and often personal, this one single factor wraps around human nature with snake-like passion.

As a manifestation of generalized anxiety disorder or as a consequence of trauma, both emotional and physical (termed Post-Traumatic Stress Disorder), stress has an obvious psychological connotation to it. The mind buckles under pressure. A sense of hopelessness swoons in.

George Libman Engel can help us better understand this tumultuous state of mind. This American psychiatrist, who spent most of his working days at the University of Rochester Medical Center in Rochester, New York, founded the biopsychosocial model, which to my mind forms the most comprehensive and scientific viewpoint on a disease state. He encompasses all three facets of modern science as prime necessities of a disease manifestation. Genetic and biochemical factors that fall under the canopy of biological attributes play as much of a role as mood, personality, and behavioral traits do as psychological factors. When coupled with social factors, such as medical issues, socioeconomic causes, familial traits, and cultural peculiarities, a complete disease state emerges. A seamless interaction between one's own biology, society, and psyche eventually forms a firm disease outline.

What then happens when you drown in a sense of hopelessness? Engel called this "the giving-up-given-up complex."

The following traits emerge:

1. A feeling of a block or an impasse from which there is no respite.
2. Poor self-image, a gross underestimation of one's own capabilities.
3. A thorough lack of gratification in terms of minimal job satisfaction or family rewards.
4. A complete breakdown of past, present, and future, with an overwhelming influence of negative thoughts oozing from the past, forming a compulsive, brooding pattern of thought process.

Another American psychologist, Lawrence LeShan, from Roosevelt University and the New York School of Social Research, probed the various phases of hopelessness. According to LeShan, hopelessness is, as an initial phase, a reflection of an individual's early experiences, beliefs, and thought patterns. The second phase is an acceptance—a vacuous obedience to any challenges, coarse or fine, a nonchalance that shows no ingenuity and no innovation, and frequently beguiles a phlegmatic façade. The third and final phase is a termination, a yielding, a giveaway to anything that was once worthwhile, be it a job or a relationship, resulting in a final sinking into the quiet waters of helplessness—a total negativity that holds sway over the individual's aptitude toward life.

LeShan categorized them into the following beliefs:

1. A stone set conviction that none can bring any help,
2. A ceaseless quagmire where no change is possible or allowed, and a constant cloud cover where no sunshine is permissible.
3. A dark sense of dogmatism that the solitary feeling of hopelessness would persist even if change is enforced.

These are situations that cry out for help. Yet they persist—in an almost surreal way—only at the indulgence of the victim, caught in the trappings of a hopeless mind that convinces itself that this is a situation destined to persist. With no solution. Somehow, with all emotions squeezed back, the stressed-out individual continues to dine out, drive to work, watch TV, and carry out virtually all activities of daily living.

Yet this is also the situation that deepens any physical ailment. Not only is the mind jolted, but the physical component also gets dented. A disease becomes a crisis when the mind crashes.

There is an outpouring of literature on these correlations. LeShan gave a disturbing example concerning this mind-body crash. When he had approached a lady named Jenny, bedridden with terminal cancer, she had said in a deathly quiet tone, "Well, I am not surprised at it, because from the beginning I had a feeling that there was no hope for me and I would never have real happiness in life."

This brings us into the hands of Aaron Beck. Considered the father of cognitive therapy, with pioneering research in psychotherapy, psychopathology, suicide, and psychometrics, Dr. Beck proposed the *negative triad*. As an irrational and pessimistic view of the three key elements of a person's belief system, the triad consists of "automatic, spontaneous, and seemingly uncontrollable negative thoughts" about the self, the world or environment, and the future.

From this concept hatched two major advancements in psychiatry: the scales for hopelessness and anxiety, as well as for the essence of cognitive therapy. As a 20-item self-report inventory, a type of psychological test in which a person fills out a survey or questionnaire with or without the help of an investigator, it was designed to measure three major aspects of hopelessness: feelings about the future, loss of motivation, and expectations. Some of the major questions included:

- ✦ I might as well give up because there's nothing I can do to make things better for me.
- ✦ I happen to be particularly lucky and I expect to get more of the good things in life than the average person.

✦ I never get what I want, so it's foolish to want anything.

✦ My past experiences have prepared me well for my future.

While stress management rolls out from every corner of the media, the crux of the problem seems as much an individual event as one caused by the environment. In other words, while environment does play a role in creating stress, individuals also exist as either prone or immune to it. And here is where scientists are flexing their muscles.

The glucocorticoid or cortisol (the naturally produced steroid hormones in response to stress) component of stress response has been the darling of all scientific research. Excess exposure to this hormone coming out of a stress-related incident has far-reaching and often ominous effects on the human system, including, but not restricted to, mood, anxiety, and cognitive aberration, including Alzheimer's. In a recent study from Johns Hopkins Hospital, differences specific and peculiar to an individual's genetic constitution have been shown to be responsible for varied glucocorticoid responses.

A neurotransmitter called dopamine dominates the other alternative. Research studies from Harvard Medical School's affiliate McLean Hospital have identified dopamine as the primary source of all these ordeals. Scientists here are predicting dopamine as the trigger for the release of the Cortisol Releasing Factor (CRF), the main chemical responsible for the flood of emotional and organic responses. More significant are the indications that early childhood exposure to abuse, stress, or trauma can bring forth such a breakdown of normal dopamine-CRF interactions.

So what happens when we are stressed out?

Things traverse well beyond the psychiatric perimeter when stress becomes an inescapable environment. From parental and/or peer pressures to professional pressures, we are one hapless bunch of *Homo sapiens* condemned to stress.

But it doesn't always come out as a hair-tearing event. Manifestations could be far more subtle, and therefore indulged. They could come as diurnal headaches, inexplicable fatigue, insomnia, restlessness, and dwindling sexual drive. Vague chest tightness, air hunger, and sweaty extremities are some of the other physical outlets. These, along with emotional and mental aberrations, are the sine qua non of a stressful attack. An oscillating distracted mind that is irascible, pessimistic, and unsure is most likely stressed out unless proven otherwise.

Dr. Beck's Anxiety Inventory is timely and pertinent. First published in the *Journal of Consulting and Clinical Psychology* in 1988, it proposed a twenty-one-question, multiple-choice, self-report inventory to measure various shades of anxiety.

With the presentation of stress being so protean, it will be worthwhile to examine the entirety of Dr. Beck's questionnaire:

+ Presence of tingling and numbness.
+ Sensation of feeling hot.
+ Wobbliness in legs.
+ Inability to relax.
+ Fear of the worst happening.
+ Dizziness or lightheadedness.
+ Pounding or racing heart.
+ Unsteadiness.
+ Feeling of terror.
+ Nervousness.
+ choking sensation,
+ Trembling hands.
+ Shakiness.
+ Fear of losing control.
+ Difficulty breathing.

✦ Feelings of fear or being scared.

✦ Indigestion or discomfort in abdomen.

✦ Fear of dying.

✦ Sensation of fainting.

✦ Flushed face.

✦ Sweating (not due to heat).

Based on responses, each question carried various points. Scores were then interpreted accordingly as:

✦ 0–7: minimal anxiety

✦ 8–15: mild anxiety

✦ 16–25: moderate anxiety

✦ 26–63: severe anxiety

But as we know, numbers may not reveal the diagnosis. I personally have noticed an all-or-nothing phenomenon in a good number of my stressed-out patients. Either they will barge in, trembling with anxiety, where Beck's Anxiety Inventory would be lifesaving, or they will retreat into a stealthy silence, where no scales can apply.

Pat Lucas was a perfect example. The first time I saw Pat in my clinic, she was composed, but quiet—excessively quiet. She complained of a tiredness that just would not quit. Pat was a forty-eight-year-old woman who ran two jobs in two shifts. She was recently divorced and lived with her twin sons, both in high school. I told her that she had enough on her plate to be physiologically tired, but because it was persistent, I would look for secondary causes. I ran some blood tests on her, included thyroid, Vitamin B_{12}, a complete blood count, and a metabolic panel. She requested a "booster," which I politely refused, not knowing what I was stepping into. All her blood results came back normal. Pat had no hypothyroidism, no vitamin deficiency, and no anemia.

She came back to me two months later, this time looking a bit flustered. Pat told me she now knew what was bothering her and what might be contributing to her fatigue. She had been nursing chronic lower back pain and had a burning sensation every time she passed urine. That was objective enough, I thought. But why hadn't she mentioned those signs to me in her first visit? Pat's answer was equally objective:

"It slipped my mind," she said, "as none of them were strong enough to interfere with my daily life schedule."

According to her, the pain was not the acute type that became a daily reminder. Instead, it was the gnawing, chewing type, mild and subtle, that she would almost forget to acknowledge. As for the burning sensation, it "comes and goes" and never really bothered her unless she paid serious attention to it.

On examination, she did seem to have left-flank tenderness, as she had jumped up when I pressed on that quadrant. Did Pat have a urinary tract infection? Was there a whimsical kidney stone that flared up once in a while? Was the urinary burning sensation a subsequence of bacteria that colonized on the stone? I found every reason to order a urinary analysis and a culture. So as not to miss anything, I also ordered a renal ultrasound. Pat did not want any medication, and I advised her to drink plenty of fluids and report to the ER in case the pain escalated.

As you are guessing by now, her urine analysis, culture, and ultrasound came out squeaky clean. Her third visit came at least six months later. She seemed agitated this time, complaining that I had not been able to get to the root of the problem. She further stated that she had been nursing a constant, band-like headache that refused to go away. Was Pat malingering? Was she a hypochondriac? Was she seeking drugs? All three were possible. But what was also possible was that Pat was suffering from stress—which she actually was. She opened up the moment I gently probed into her personal life. A raging, tumultuous friction in her life had been tormenting her ever since her divorce. Not one to pine for something that was lost, Pat had put up a brave front. She wanted to desperately scuttle her past thoughts, a distracting wistfulness, unworthy of nostalgia. She countered them with work, work, and more work. In the process, she felt exhausted and drained. Worse, her body started to reject the enforced burden and protested with back pain, fatigue, and tension-type headaches.

Are we genetically destined to be stressed out?

There are no absolute right answers. While propensities cannot be denied, there is every opportunity to come out of it. Medications exist. However, many, many other non-pharmaceutical management options are on the menu, too. Realizing the disastrous potential of continued stress on the heart and mind, health research has come out with numerous coping exercises. These could be imperative basics, such as asking for help or talking to a therapist. Self-governed techniques, including exercising, watching movies, listening to relaxation tapes, vacationing, and cultivating hobbies, are all external resources that are momentary but vital to the burned-out soul.

The bottom line remains the need for an effective *channelization* to an area of internal comfort that can blunt the potential trigger and effectively bring down the damaging effects of the springing steroids. Along with channelization comes a firm realization that true contentment is a fiercely independent character.

LeShan proposed that an individual should first accept his or her own being as valid and seek inner fulfillment. Where would the fulfillment come from? The belief that any and all lives have a meaningful purpose becomes the inner source of fulfillment—that there is a road for every traveler and a shelter for every seeker—a personal star to look up to, no matter from what distance they twinkle.

Stress, Alzheimer's Dementia, and Yoga

But what does stress have to do with Alzheimer's?

This is a million-dollar question that psychiatrist Dr. Linda Mah from the University of Toronto answered from her neuroscience lab. Leading a Canadian team, Dr. Mah found that stress, conceptualized as an adaptive response to a specific challenge, adversely affects three critical areas of the brain: amygdala, Prefrontal Cortex (PFC), and hippocampus.

The eye of the storm fell on the hippocampus because not only does it play a vital role in memory formation; it also serves to regulate emotions by relaying *contextual* information about a specific threat through its interaction with the amygdala and PFC. In normal situations, the hippocampus allows an individual to discriminate between threat and safety.

To summarize and simplify, the amygdala functions to detect threat and generate emotional responses, such as fear and anxiety. By contrast, the hippocampus and the medial prefrontal cortex (mPFC) down-regulate to tame those excesses. In grand harmony, this balance creates an emotional equivalence between the amygdala and the dual action of the hippocampus and PFC. Dr. Mah and her team proved that stress completely destroys this balance by reversing the thermostat of our emotional equilibrium.

Pooling data from studies of lab animals, human brain scans, and the damaging effects of excessive catecholamine and cortisol, which are released during stressful events, the researchers went on to demonstrate effectively a disorganized, exaggerated amygdala activity failing to govern emotional responses and the structural degeneration of the hippocampus and PFC that failed to regulate those responses through thinking.

What conclusion was reached from these demonstrations?

According to Dr. Mah, "Pathological anxiety and chronic stress are associated with structural degeneration and impaired functioning of the hippocampus and the prefrontal cortex (PFC), which may account for the increased risk of developing neuropsychiatric disorders, including depression, and dementia."

The lab's work suggested that by reducing chronic stress by therapy, exercise or mindfulness meditation, one should be able to reduce the risk of Alzheimer's.

"Looking into the future," said Dr. Mah, "we need to do more work to determine whether interventions, such as exercise, mindfulness training, and cognitive behavioral therapy, can not only reduce stress but decrease the risk of developing neuropsychiatric disorders."

Returning again to Harvard University, one can appreciate yoga's tremendous résumé. The institution is replete with the management of stress through the ancient practice of yoga and meditation. Dr. Ann Webster, health psychologist at the Benson-Henry Institute for Mind-Body Medicine at the Harvard-affiliated Massachusetts General Hospital, cuts no corners when it comes to defining the ill effects of stress.

"As we age," Dr. Webster says, "our immune systems are less efficient, and adding stress to that can lead to disease progression or the onset of disease."

Regarding stress management, she is equally objective. Along with Cognitive Behavioral Therapy, she strongly emphasizes the rewards of relaxation techniques, such as yoga, meditation, guided imagery, and deep-breathing exercises. As triggers of relaxation response, the effects are physiological, involving the lowering of blood pressure, heart rate, respiratory rate, oxygen consumption, and stress hormones.

This is the essential strength and beauty of yoga. It takes a step beyond external calming resources. With its integral, inherent potential, it quiets the storm from within and converts the rebel into a rational, thinking mind with a mastery that has neither the adverse effects nor the resistance of a commercial compound.

Yoga for Caregivers

In most instances, caregivers go unnoticed and unseen. Helping hands are meant to be strong and healthy, and if they are not, they need replacement. The scientific world has had little patience or shown little interest in delving into the psyche of caregivers. Unfortunately, very few scientists have come forward to highlight such unnoticed suffering.

In 2004, L. C. Waelde and his colleagues conducted a pilot study on twelve women taking care of relatives who were giving care to demented patients. The pilot utilized a program called Inner Resources that included meditation, yoga postures (*asanas*), breathing techniques, and repetition of specific sounds (*mantras*). Specific questionnaires filled out by the caregivers following the program revealed considerable improvements in their state of anxiety and depression.

Eight years later, authors K. E. Innes, A. Thompson-Heisterman, and others, undertook research on the effects of meditation on stress and related indices of psychological status on both demented patients and their caregivers. Despite their informative conclusions that showed the benefits of meditation, both studies lacked statistical power, owing to the very small number of participants and lack of controls.

In the same year (2012), a statistically stronger study rolled out from the Department of Psychobiology at the Universidade Federal de São Paolo in Brazil. Scientists M. A. D. Danucalov, J. R. Leite and others focused on forty-six familial caregivers of patients with Alzheimer's disease. While one group of twenty-five random volunteers underwent a yoga and compassion program for eight weeks, the remaining participants served as the control. The researchers used three standard instruments to measure the outcomes:

1. The Lipp's Stress Symptoms Inventory for Adults (LSSI), a stress detection set that was very popular in Brazil, and based

its results on a four-phase model of alertness, resistance, qua-
siexhaustion, and exhaustion.

2. The standard Beck Depression (BDI) and Beck Anxiety Inventory (BAI), described earlier and universally adopted.

3. Salivary cortisol level.

The scientists pursued familiar targets: stress, anxiety, depression,
and morning salivary cortisol levels. All four showed a dramatic
decrease in participants who underwent the yoga and meditation
program. So as not to disappoint the biostatisticians, all reductions
showed statistical significance.

Yoga's Endless Repertoire

We have not as yet unveiled the full rewards available from yoga.
What we have unearthed thus far seems to offer a life that can become
sublime in depth and quality. A look at the *Harvard Health Publication* from the Harvard Medical School provides a bird's-eye view of
how advanced and prolific yoga's journey has become.

Titled as "Yoga: Health Benefits Beyond the Mat," this publication
carries the following informations for patients:

Better Body Image: Focusing inward during yoga helps you be
more satisfied with and less critical of your body.

Heart Benefits: Yoga can lower blood pressure, cholesterol, and
blood sugar.

Overall Fitness: Yoga increases muscle strength and flexibility,
boosts endurance, and tunes up heart, lungs, and blood vessels.

Mindful Eating: Being aware of how your body feels carries over
to mealtimes.

Weight Control: Mindfulness developed through yoga can make
you more sensitive to cues of hunger and fullness.

Results from various studies from other universities have been gratifying, to say the least. One marvels at yoga's prodigious reach. It has been shown to improve cardiovascular and respiratory functions, and both physical and mental health. At a more fundamental level, research has found that yoga decreases the sympathetic tone (a part of the autonomic nervous system that increases heart rate), and constricts blood vessels to increase blood pressure (the so-called Adrenaline rush), while encouraging the parasympathetic tone with an anticipated opposite calming effect, which is necessary to combat stress and strain.

This is not a catharsis or purge of stress factors, but rather a heightened power to absorb and channelize the same.

Helen Lavretsky, professor at the University of California in Los Angeles, walked an extra mile. She led a group of scientists to research twenty-five participants, some of whom received memory enhancement training and other practical strategies of memory training, while the rest took a three-month course on two specific types of yoga: Kirtan Kriya and Kundalini Yoga, both involving a series of exercises, breathing, and *mantras*. Both behavioral changes and brain activities were measured.

According to Dr. Lavretsky, "Memory training was comparable to yoga with meditation in terms of improving memory, but yoga provided a broader benefit than memory training because it also helped with mood, anxiety, and coping skills."

Case Studies: Indispensable Hands of Yoga in Mass Casualties

The Tsunami Disaster

Call it ambivalence, dichotomy, or downright unpredictability—our world understands the absurdity of balance. On December 25, 2004, as three quarters of the world basked in the solemn joy of yet another Christmas, few knew of the horror that would follow over the next few hours.

The exquisite silence of a sacred night had little clue of an onrushing storm, brewing only inches away. An underprepared part of the world had little anticipation of earth's tectonic plates colliding far beneath. Such was the terrifying innocence and ignorance that as a distant earthquake seduced the ocean waters of Sumatra's Aceh Province, children danced on the beach, blissfully unaware that twenty minutes later, swirling waters would bludgeon the land, leaving humanity with little to no chance of survival.

Death dominated on December 26, as hundreds of thousands disappeared in nature's one decisive sweep. What emerged from the death and destruction were despair and desolation. Stress, depression, and isolation invaded every remaining mind huddled in camps and makeshift settlements.

While financial and physical support poured in from all quarters of the world, the United Nations, among others, offered emotional guidance to those reeling under relentless agony and stress. When Dr. Patricia L. Gerbarg from New York Medical College, Valhalla, and Dr. Richard P. Brown from Columbia University's College of Physicians and Surgeons in New York, heard that the International Association for Human Values, a United Nations NGO, was delivering yoga programs to thousands of survivors of the tsunami, they readily offered to study the effects.

Collaborating with the Trauma Resolution Center of Miami, the National Institute of Mental Health and Neurosciences of India, and Ved Vignan Maha Vidya Peeth (VVMVP) of Bangalore, India, the scientists planned a randomized controlled study of an eight-hour, breath-based yoga program, called Breath Water Sound (BWS), enhanced with *sudarshan kriya* (a Sanskrit term depicting an advanced form of rhythmic, cyclical breathing, with slow, medium, and fast cycles), and an exposure therapy, called Trauma Incident Reduction (TIR).

Developed by Sri Sri Ravi Shankar, founder of the Art of Living, the world's most comprehensive yoga family, Breath Water Sound included *ujjayi* and *bhastrika* (bellows) breathing techniques. The ten-minute *sudarshan kriya* consisted of cyclical breathing at slow, medium, and fast rates.

This entire twenty-four-week study had both the challenges and chills of an edge-of-the-seat thriller. VVMVP provided yoga teachers and Tamil-speaking volunteers. One of the teachers, Teresa Descilo, trained and supervised the testers and TIR facilitators. B. Damodaran, a local inhabitant who was familiar with local customs, organized and supervised the on-site study. The team focused on 183 tsunami survivors from the most severely devastated coastal villages, who were still living in five refugee camps eight months after the tsunami.

The refugee camp administrator offered the primary challenge. Randomization, the hallmark of any scientific study where groups receiving or not receiving yoga benefits are randomly assigned, was thrown out of the contest. The administrator was afraid that it would spark controversy and protests among survivors as unfair treatment, thereby disrupting the social order of the camp. The first compromise ensured that entire camps were assigned to each group, rather than being strictly randomized.

The second challenge came from the refugees, themselves. Buried in a quicksand of ignorance, they had neither the knowledge nor the basic concept to carry out any instructions pertinent to a trial. Damodaran was afraid they would fail to keep their benefits to themselves and would "shout out answers and invalidate the tests." This meant that an army of testers was needed to test each participant individually. This was a Herculean task by any means, as a total of 2,500 tests were individually administered by testers sitting in heat exceeding 100 degrees for more than 800 person-hours.

Confidentiality and gender bias presented the greatest challenge. The scientists were performing research in a part of the world where discussions of sexuality or sexual preferences were not openly artic-ulated. The last question on the Beck Depression Inventory, asking about sexual desire, had to be dropped, denting the test's validity. Despite that omission, the confidential questionnaires provided unex-pected opportunities for many females to speak about the frequent abuses they had to withstand, including one woman who revealed that her brother-in-law had repeatedly raped her. The unbearable stress burdening her came not from Mother Nature, but from home.

One particular incident during this time stood out as extraor-dinary and almost surreal, yet medically plausible if viewed in the right context. As a part of Somatic Symptom Disorder, conversion disorder (a psychiatric condition that cannot be explained by medical evaluation) has various expressions. This is diagnosed when people have neurological symptoms that cannot be traced back to a medical cause. For example, patients may have the following symptoms:

+ Weakness or paralysis.
+ Abnormal movements (such as tremor or unsteady gait).
+ Blindness.
+ Hearing loss.
+ Loss of sensation, or numbness.

While Damodaran was deeply engaged in his work, he heard a hissing sound, along with a shout from one of the facilitators. Periph-erally, he saw a woman looking at him from the window, eyes rolled back in a blank stare, her tongue forking out, her wriggling body crawling on all fours, bent as a sickle. This was a complete conversion of a woman to a snake-like contour, with snake-like movement, and a snake-like attitude. Damodaran confronted her and calmed her. She was breathing heavily and rapidly. Slowly but surely, as she molted out of her snake-self, a bitter story unfolded—a story of relentless stress and emotional abuse from her mother-in-law. Quietly surrendering to these unyielding abusive diatribes, her subconscious unconditionally surrendered to a snake-like state.

Damodaran listened to her story, allowing the acid to trickle out from her emotions. He worked with her on slow-breathing techniques and placed her in the same eight-hour breath-based yoga program involving the rest of the sufferers from the tsunami.

The common denominator for all was stress.

A Post-Traumatic Checklist (PCL-17) was used to measure the stressful emotions. Those who scored more than fifty were assigned by the camps to one of three groups: yoga-breath intervention (BWS); yoga-breath intervention, followed by three to eight hours of trauma-reduction exposure technique (BWS + TIR), or a six-week wait-list.

Both PCL (for stress) and BDI (for depression) scores were used to tabulate the changes in the ensuing weeks. The results of the eight-week program were unequivocal and decisive. After six weeks, decreases of at least 60 percent in mean scores on the PCL-17 and 90 percent on the BDI occurred in the groups given BWS alone and BWS + TIR, compared to no change in the control group. In the BWS group, most of the improvement occurred within the first week. The benefits were maintained at a twenty-four-week follow-up.

It included, most gratifyingly, our abused lady. She went back to confront her earthly challenges, shedding both her snake-like existence and her overwhelming depression.

The Rwandan Genocide

One of the most grotesque dichotomies ever shown was featured on the front page of *The New York Times*, in two pictures placed side by side. The left frame carried the jubilant Brazilian soccer players after they won the 1994 World Cup. The right frame depicted skulls, one brushing the other, neatly stacked, and belonging to men, women, and children of the Tutsi clan who were slaughtered by the Hutu majority of Rwanda.

No other piece of reported information could match the brittleness of human emotions as did those two pictures. What nature did in a tsunami, men accomplished even more evilly, and purposefully, in the Rwandan genocide. An estimated 500,000 to 1,000,000 Rwandans were killed during the 100-day period from early April to mid-July 1994, constituting as many as 70 percent of the Tutsi and 20 percent of Rwanda's total population. As expected, helpless to the trail of mass murders, rapes, and torture, countless more sank into abject stress, depression, and agony. Such was the physical pain of the very annihilation, that little help was sought to heal the minds that were left behind in complete tatters.

It took more than a decade to reach those minds. Founded in 2004 to promote Conscious Social Change for women and girls, Global Grassroots was custom-made for Rwanda and other post-conflict countries. In 2006, the organization reached out to those who stood and suffered on the burning deck of their life.

Rape, abuse, and torture—all had been hurled at them.

They had escaped death, but embraced all that was defined by it while living—a limitless vacuum that only harbored hopelessness. Much later, in 2010, during the International Symposium on the Genocide Perpetrated Against Tutsi, the Ministry of Health reported that "80 percent of Rwandese experienced trauma during the genocide, and today 28.5 percent of Rwandese still have symptoms of PTSD, over 50 percent of whom also present with comorbid depression."

What exactly is Conscious Social Change as proposed by this nonprofit organization? The official website describes it succinctly as "the intersection of mindfulness, leadership, and social entrepreneurship whereby individuals may initiate change consciously, compassionately, and ethically."

And what was offered to those hapless victims, especially to the traumatized women? Essentially breath work, mindfulness, meditation, and deep listening.

In the first two weeks, these women learned daily mind-body practices, including gentle Hatha Yoga, guided meditation, mindfulness, somatic exercises, and other holistic approaches. None of this was easy, despite being intended to help. These were not to be attractive yoga postures, fashioned in dim-lit studios. The teachers knew and appreciated that their students were victims of rape and abuse, standing at the brink of emotional collapse. In fact, studies have shown that 79 percent of these cohorts of PTSD patients surfaced their occult emotions during the annual genocide commemoration period.

Researchers also knew that in Rwanda, they were looking at a completely different cultural and linguistic challenge. In fact, in that country's language, there existed no terminology or words reflecting the phrase Post-Traumatic Stress Disorder (PTSD). A new word, *Gahukamuka*, had to be invented "to encompass experiences related to the genocide, including despair, excessive crying, being easily startled, having flashbacks, and repeatedly dreaming of bad events." Furthermore, victims in Rwanda were made to lie down side by side prior to execution, which meant that those who survived continued to suffer from bristling sensitivity to any condition that recalled that ill-fated supine posture. Any yoga pose that remotely resembled lying down had to be discarded.

Despite all these regional and personal restraints, the interventions paid rich dividends. All who responded to the mind-body portion of the questionnaire found value in personal consciousness practices. The women successfully adapted them to their daily needs.

A meaningful life had finally broken free of the cobwebs of relentless despair and depression.

Fueled by the success of the tsunami survivors, researchers adopted similar yoga and breath techniques, resulting in positive outcomes in other natural disasters, such as the 2010 Haiti earthquakes and manmade disasters, such as post-war Sudan in 2010.

Mind-Body Program: A Safe Haven

The two examples included here—the tsunami disaster and the Rwandan genocide—demonstrate the benefits of yoga in flinging open a brand-new window of hope and healing for the management of mass disasters, whether created by nature or man. Whatever the entry gates, in contrast to an isolated event, mass disasters carry within them far-reaching and persistent consequences. In other words, over and above the instant effects of any suffering, the potential of disorder harboring long after the happening is agonizingly viable in any global-scale disaster. In many ways, they parallel the effects of chronic diseases, such as cancer, a debilitating stroke, or any terminal illness, where mental and emotional challenges linger and frequently overshadow physical disabilities.

As we have seen, generic prescriptions of antidepressants or anxiolytics fall woefully short of any meaningful cure. By the word *meaningful* I mean any mental or emotional challenges that withstand the hands of time. Especially in mass-scale disaster situations, it is not feasible to shower pills on a community. At best, one can subdue an upheaval but not nullify its existence. Drugs save lives, but rarely uproot a cause. At best, we as providers can procrastinate the proceedings, suppress the exhibitions, and keep the inevitable at bay.

As a part of the mind-body system, this then becomes yoga's claim to a comprehensive cure. Not as an external resource, but more as an internal realignment of a system that has been disturbed. For the long-term effects of an untoward event, an integral approach becomes a refuge, not just a relief.

What are the benefits of mind-body programs from a pragmatic standpoint?

There are more than many. First, unlike a drug treading on unknown bodies, these programs carry the flexibility to adapt to the local needs, cultures, religions, and even languages of a particular geographical area. We are looking at breathing techniques, postures, and meditation skills, all three of which are refreshingly independent of any culture, religion, or societal taste—exclusive, and yet universal.

Second, not being enmeshed in a pharmaceutically-driven product or dependent on coverage from insurance companies, these programs are instantly accessible and low-cost, requiring no equipment, electricity, or specific spaces. Not even a crowd of health professionals is needed! These programs can reach out to community leaders who themselves become the vanguards of these holistic movements. They can be trained to learn, and teach the basics of breath techniques and postures to the victims or sufferers. These benefits assume priceless proportions when one keeps in mind that these psychological effects can trespass, unperturbed, for endless miles, affecting subsequent generations.

Pat Lucas, my stressed-out patient, did not want any yoga or meditation. She had little time for "such cults." She wanted a quick fix, and preferred Xanax. When I refused to refill her pills on her return visit, she walked away. I haven't heard from her since.

I still hope that she will return one day and embrace a more profound avenue of care.

5

MEDITATION AND YOGA: THE BUILDING BLOCKS

*Not even the deepest sleep will give you
such a rest as meditation can.*

—Swami Vivekananda

I t's been more than thirty years since I first encountered meditation as a boy. Yet despite the ensuing years of heat and dust, those moments remain crystal clear, resonating with star-like clarity under a peach-blue sky.

As a young lad of barely ten years, walking three miles was like crossing the street. My journey from home to the temple where I practiced meditation was a thirty-minute affair, something that I happily indulged. The sun would invariably retire by the time I entered the entrance of the Gol Park Institute of Culture, lodged in perfect serenity amid the swirling traffic of India's South Calcutta.

I loved to meditate. One could almost feel the chaos of a bustling city hungering for a spot of silence. But that was not the real reason. In

India, meditation is practically a sport, a passion like soccer, basketball, cricket, and other forms of entertainment. Every god sits in the meditative pose. Meditation is taught in school, cultured in scholarly circles, and endorsed by health professionals. Even the communists meditate by default. It cuts across state borders, religious proclivities, and political ideologies. It is India's one solitary baton that is naturally and ceaselessly passed along.

Even today, my back can feel the soft, padded palm of the monk. That was the first step of meditation I was taught—to sit straight, with a fluent, unbent spine that would ceaselessly connect the sacrum to the atlas.

"This will create the right platform for the right type of breathing."

The monk spoke almost in an undertone as he straightened the thoracic curve of my spine. Years later, as a medical student, I learned the outstanding benefits of sitting straight. Slouching may not give a person a hunchback overnight. But if slouched every day on weak, sagging muscles, the whole skeletal framework can change. Much later in my clinical days, I realized chronic low-back pain as an inevitable outcome of a slouched and bent spine.

According to Mladen Golubic, Medical Director for the Center for Lifestyle Medicine at Cleveland Clinic's Wellness Institute, perfect posture is relaxed and straight, with a core of strong shoulder blades active but not tight, and with an erect spine. The results, as Dr. Golubic says, "expands your chest, allowing you to take in a larger breath . . . and you will have more energy and focus." It comes as little surprise that he almost always advises his patients to start yoga. "The first thing we learn in yoga is how to sit properly."

What, then, are we proposing to achieve through yoga?

Let me hop, skip, and jump over all scholarly interpretations and go directly to the fundamental remarks Patanjali made thousands of years ago. According to this wise man, yoga is essentially a "subjugation of the thought waves of the mind."

The tempting simile is that of a lake. A thin film of water knows no language other than restlessness touching its surface. Anything and everything blows across its mind, from a pebble tossed to the slightest breeze. The gentle ripples are not waves that heave and thrash. Instead, they ruffle the surface constantly and incessantly.

This is our mind, helpless to the unending procession of our thoughts touching it from all around. The bed that lies at the very bottom of the lake is our unrealized self—completely unrecognized, covered and clouded by those ripples.

Yoga's primary objective is to un-ripple the thin watery surface, to smooth out the wrinkles, and still the waters, like a transparent mirror through which the bed can be seen and felt. When personified, yoga controls the outgoing tendencies of the mind, the senses, and the body. It calls for regulated practice and discipline. An eightfold system of practice is employed. Sequentially, one process falls into the other:

Restraint
Discipline
Posture (*asana*)
Control of breath (*pranayama*)
Withdrawal of the mind
Concentration
Meditation
Absorption

The first five steps should be self-explanatory. The last three make for interesting applications.

We will concentrate on these eight processes. As we proceed, it will be prudent for us to bear in mind that Patanjali, and subsequently Buddha, maintained strong spiritual connotations at every step of their yoga practice. Refreshingly, they steered clear of any dogmatic rituals that could define a particular religion. Instead, yoga and its principles preached virtues that were holistic and omnipresent. Unlike a church or temple or mosque, there was no curved canopy heralding a man sitting under the tree in a lotus position. Buddha simply spoke about fundamental paths of life in utter simplicity, devoid of any rigid constitution.

We will honor the simplistic fundamentals of life as we address the eightfold system of a *Yogi*.

1. Restraint (*yama*): Here, yoga calls for the cultivation of five virtues: nonviolence, truthfulness, non-covetousness, continence, and non-receiving of gifts and favors.
2. Discipline (*niyama*): This process constitutes five observances: cleanliness, contentment, austerity, repetition of sacred words (mantras), and surrendering the fruits of all action to the divine.
3. Posture (*asana*): This is supremely important and calls for precision because of the tremendous emphasis yoga lays on its correctness. At a basic level, the limbs of the body should be in a restful state that is conducive to concentration and meditation. The meditator sits straight and erect, with a spinal cord that is unbent, yet relaxed. The idea is to hold the back, neck, and head in a straight continuity, with the entire weight of the upper body resting on the ribs.

In his Aphorisms, Patanjali describes correct posture as one that is "firm and pleasant."

To quote Vivekananda:

"Firmness of posture means that you do not feel the body at all. Generally speaking, you will find that as soon as you sit for a few minutes you feel all sorts of bodily disturbances. But when you have gone beyond the idea of a gross, physical body, you will lose all sense of the body. You will feel neither pleasure nor pain. And when you again become aware of it, you will feel completely rested. This is the only real rest that you can give to the body. When you have succeeded in controlling the body and keeping it firm, your practice will be steady, but while you are disturbed by the body, your nerves become disturbed and you cannot concentrate on the mind."

Yogic postures number approximately 84, yet only a few entail meditation as part of them. Of these, the one that stands out as popular, adoptable, and of immense benefit is the *padmasana*, or lotus position. Technique-wise, the practitioner sits with legs crossed, each foot resting sole up on the opposite thigh. The spinal column up to the base of the brain is held completely erect. Hands are placed in the lap with palms up, one hand on top of the other with thumbs touching. The other option is to place the hands on the thighs. The eyes are traditionally kept half open, with attention focused either on the heart or between the eyebrows.

What are the watch words for any *asana* (posture)?

+ A posture that is firm and pleasant.
+ Seated motionlessly and comfortably, with eyes half closed to half open, beyond external and internal distractions.
+ An alignment that is continuous from brain to base, with a straight, free-flowing spine.
+ Control of breath (*pranayama*). This is another pivotal point of practice, which I will return to in greater detail. To the yoga system, our breath is a part of the cosmic energy (*prana*). A regulated and a harmonious breath calms the mind.
+ Withdrawal of mind (*pratyahara*). An art that invokes serious discipline and training to detach itself at will from each sense organ. To my mind, this forms the first hushed steps into the meditative state.

✦ Concentration (*dhyana*). You will notice by now how logically each step eases into the next. Once the art of withdrawing is addressed, the art of keeping the mind focused on an object for a certain length of time, without any disjunction, is the next to be mastered.

✦ Meditation (*dhyana*): This, then, is the crux of the process—a state of effortless and continuous concentration, "like the flow of oil poured from one vessel into another." The yoga system recognizes five cardinal levels of the mind:

1. Dull and stupefied.
2. Restless and turbulent.
3. Distracted and divided.
4. Concentrated and one-pointed.
5. Restrained and suspended.

The first three states of mind are not conducive to the art of meditation.

To quote Patanjali:

"Meditation is the uninterrupted concentration of thought on its object. This itself turns into Samadhi when the object alone shines and the thought of meditation (and of the meditator) is lost, as it were."

Absorption (*samadhi*): The climax is reached when meditation is constant and continuous, and the mind merges into the object of meditation.

Before we attempt to unravel the basic building blocks of meditation, we must ask ourselves a fundamental question.

What is a best time to meditate? Or is there an appropriate moment to meditate?

To the retired and the relaxed, this is hardly a challenging question. To the working parent or college student, however, this can be impossible to answer—and even worse for the doctor working alternate day and night shifts. Ideally, from the spiritual point of view—and scientifically, too—moments of complete tranquility are most conducive. In meditation, we are talking about attention, perception, and concentration—open or focused. Silence is the language you want to hear and be heard by spiritual souls. Globally, and across all religions, you would choose the crack of dawn, a time of enchantment only nature provides.

Vivekananda makes a poignant statement:

> "What is the best time for practice in yoga? The junction time of dawn and twilight, when all nature becomes calm. Take the help of nature."

But how about the college student, studying late hours and sleeping like a baby in the wee hours of the morning? How about the nurse, exhausted after a long night of uninterrupted care and service? The solution lies in finding silence—anytime and anywhere, away from the screams of the outside world, in a comfortable corner.

When it comes to Transcendental Meditation, the entire process of internalization rests on the *mantra*, the sound or word that is repeatedly uttered. Every religious being will attest that there exists a key word or phrase in his or her religion that generates tremendous power—be it in faith or in fervor.

Just as *Lord Jesus Christ, Son of God, have mercy on me* encompasses all that is pure and powerful to Christians, so does *Barukh Atab Adonai* to followers of Judaism and *Bismillah ir-Rahman ir Rahim* to devotees of Islam.

The word *Om* from the ancient Veda has similarly transcended time and space to be used for peace and gratification. The classical *Gayatri Mantra*, as it occurs in the *Rig Veda*, reads as follows in Sanskrit:

Om. Bhur Buvah Shah
Tat Savitur-Varenyam
Bhargo Devasya Dhimahi
Dhio Yo Nah Prachodayat. Om

In short, the mantra recognizes the sun, the visible luminary in the sky, as the reflection of the Supreme Being. The seeker meditates on that light, as the light of absolute reality. From a practical standpoint, while meditating on the *Gayatri mantra*, the meditator is required to direct attention to the radiance of the sunlight and then contemplate inwards to perceive the source of light within. In an advanced stage, the identity of the light inside and the light of the sun are appreciated as the Pure Consciousness of the inner self, the all-pervading Pure Consciousness of the universal Self.

Pranayam:
The Art of Harnessing Your Breath

The technical intricacies of the practices of meditation and yoga are best left to certified teachers and seasoned practitioners. However, basic postures and breath control have weathered the test of time and emerged as fundamentals to be mastered in one's bedroom with relative comfort and ease. While supervision at its inception is recommended, the user-friendly, uncomplicated approaches of the facets of both techniques preclude strict institutional guidance.

It is relevant and prudent to mention here that *pranayama* at its deepest level is more than an exercise. In the spiritual context, it is not just a procedure of breathing in and out, in a controlled fashion, without any disjunctions. The technique dives into deeper waters to seek the subconscious level, a path that is fraught with physical and mental repercussions and lacks strong spiritual convictions and austere discipline.

To the seeker of a calm, harmonious, and un-stressed mind, these are roads best not traveled. For the purpose of clarity and accessibility, we will thus revert to the building blocks of breath control and take a brief sojourn into the anatomy, physiology, and mechanics of our breathing. In most cases, they are intricately entwined.

As a combination of inspiration and expiration, the one structure that plays a pivotal role in the act of respiration is the diaphragm. A dome-shaped structure that separates the thoracic and abdominal cavities, it is the cardinal muscle of inspiration. When it contracts, it travels downward and, being attached to the lower ribs, rotates them toward the horizontal plane. The intercostal muscles attached to the ribs also contract and join the dance. The inevitable result is an expansion of the chest cavity. Fresh air, brimming with oxygen, gushes in along the branching airways into the fundamental air pockets of the lungs, called alveoli, until the alveolar pressure stands equal to the pressure at the airway opening. In perfect synchrony, blood enters the lungs through the pulmonary artery, picks up the oxygen, and starts its triumphant course through our body, blessing cell after cell with its basic cry for life.

The reverse happens simultaneously as, sapped of all oxygen and energy, blood returns to the lungs, carrying the toxic carbon dioxide that will be exhaled by a thoracic cavity shrunken by the relaxing diaphragm and the intercostal muscles.

What adds to this wondrous spectacle is the observation that the movement of the diaphragm is not a fixed act. In normal, quiet breathing, it moves downward for about one centimeter, yet on forced inspiration/expiration, its total back-and-forth could add up to 10 centimeters. This assumes tremendous importance when deeper breathing is solicited, either in duress or by choice. For unlike other visceral involvements, be they gastrointestinal or cardiovascular, the act of breathing is both autonomic and voluntary.

To the *Yogi*, striving for control of his or her own breathing, these become indispensable tools to exploit. It is a gracious fact that the controlling powers of the mechanics of breathing lie in the brain, where the respiratory center in the brain stem directs the respiratory muscles. The medulla, located not far from the spinal cord, signals the spinal cord to maintain breathing, while the pons, a part of the brain located very near the medulla, provides further smoothing of the respiration pattern. The entire process is constant, continuous, and completely involuntary.

Changes occur in special situations, when demands for oxygen soar during physical or emotional challenges. Chemoreceptors located throughout all arteries, which are sensitive to the slightest of changes, send stirring instructions to the respiratory center to modify the speed and depth of breathing. In this case, a broad-minded diaphragm with its ability to cover 10 centimeters becomes priceless.

As you would expect, the brain governs the voluntary part of breathing, when if required, the cortex initiates decisions. Whether one is singing, playing the saxophone, or simply verbalizing contempt, the voluntary part of breathing modifies accordingly.

This sets the template of *pranayama*. The masters of this art control this very voluntary aspect of breathing. The word *prana* from *pranayama* has been frequently referred to as energy, or "life force." This makes sense when we take into account that the basic metabolism in our cells is an oxygen-dependent energy process. As researchers Ravinder Jerath and his colleagues working at the Augusta Women Center in Georgia learned, the basic physiological responses from *pranayama* range from the cellular to the electrical. They proposed that voluntary, slow, deep breathing, as pursued in *pranayama,* functionally resets the autonomic nervous system and drags it away from its excitatory (sympathetic) state.

This scientists observed that during *pranayama* inspiration the lung tissue stretches, producing inhibitory signals by the action of slowly adapting stretch receptors (SARs) and hyperpolarization currents, a state where the nerve is unable to generate electricity, by the action of fibroblasts. These very dual consequences of stretch-induced inhibitory signals and hyperpolarization currents synchronize the neural elements in the heart, lungs, limbic system, and cortex. The results were decisive and exactly what the *Yogi* desires to achieve through the act of *pranayama*—a modulation of the nervous system and decreased metabolic activity indicative of the parasympathetic state., creating a paradigm shift from an excitatory state to a state of sustained tranquility.

The researchers from Georgia discovered a "presence of decreased oxygen consumption, decreased heart rate, and decreased blood pressure, as well as increased theta wave amplitude in EEG recordings, increased parasympathetic activity accompanied by the experience of alertness and reinvigoration."

Let us return to the textual principles of *pranayama* as formally documented in the ancient books. Patanjali's definition of actual *pranayama* is based on ancient Vedic literature and begins when the breath is stopped for a period of time between inhalation and exhalation. It is also considered *pranayama* when the breath is held after an exhalation or before an inhalation.

Seasoned practitioners have proposed and practiced a formula. Following a ratio of 1:4:2, retention is required to be four times longer than inhalation and two times longer than exhalation. The progress of *pranayama* is reflected by the increasing duration of retention that is gradually mastered over a long period of time. Thus, the gradual increase in the ratio formula can be 2:8:4; 3:12:6; or 4:16:8.

As an illustration of the 4:16:8 formula, the following steps can be practiced:

1. Sit in a lotus posture. Using the thumb of the right hand, close the right nostril. Gently inhale through the left nostril. Count four during the process.
2. Using the third and fourth fingers of the right hand, close the left nostril. With both nostrils closed, retain the breath while counting up to sixteen.
3. Release the right nostril. Exhalation takes place, quite like the process of inhalation, gently and slowly. While exhaling, count eight, keeping the left nostril closed.
4. With the left nostril still closed and the right nostril open, inhale, counting up to four.
5. Close the right nostril. With both nostrils closed, retain the breath, counting to sixteen.
6. Release the left nostril. Exhalation follows, slowly and gently. Count up to eight, keeping the right nostril closed.
7. Return to original posture with both nostrils open.

It is important to re-emphasize that these are by no means guidelines to be imbibed without supervision, as we must respect the complexities involved in these processes. Like every art based on science, *pranayama,* and indeed the entire practice of meditation, is an individual journey that has its own, tailor-made, starting and finishing line. An asthmatic patient is a different individual than a patient with heart failure.

An inward journey of tranquility, be it through simple meditation or the practice of yoga, must be customized according to one's own physical capabilities.

Pranayama and Stress: Researched Evidence

Can these *pranayama* techniques be used to address stress?

Dr. Vivek Sharma and his colleagues from the Department of

Psychology of Jawaharlal Institute of Postgraduate Medical Education in India embarked on an ambitious study to demonstrate the effects of various types of *pranayama* breathing techniques on stress and other cardiovascular parameters.

Ninety individuals of both genders, all between eighteen and twenty-six years of age, were drafted into the study. They were randomly allocated into three groups. Under the supervision of a certified yoga trainer, Group One was trained in *fast pranayama* (a six-minute cycle of three specific types of *pranayama*, with three cycles lasting one session): Group Two received *slow pranayama* (a seven-minute cycle of specific *pranayama* techniques, with seven cycles lasting one session), and Group Three acted as controls.

The entire study lasted twelve weeks, and measured the following parameters:

+ Systolic and Diastolic Blood Pressure (SBP and DBP).
+ Mean Arterial Pressure (MAP).
+ Heart Rate (HR).
+ Rate Pressure Product (RPP calculated as {HRxSBP}/100).
+ Double Product (Do P= HRxMAP).

But how do you document stress? Unlike the vital parameters above, whose changes can be measured and graphed, stress, like any other emotional challenges, can be tricky, cursory, and notoriously subjective.

For this, the researchers turned to Sheldon Cohen, the Robert E. Doherty University Professor of Psychology at Carnegie Mellon University and the director of the Laboratory for the Study of Stress, Immunity and Disease. A pioneer in the field of stress, for the past thirty years he has studied the neuroendocrine, immune, and behavioral pathways that link stress, personality, and social networks to disease susceptibility. He and his team developed a good number of scales to address and stage stress. Some of the outstanding ones used frequently in research circles that assess psychological and social variables include the Perceived Stress Scale (PSS), the Interpersonal Support Evaluation Scale (ISEL), the Social Network Index (SNI), the Partner Interaction Questionnaire (PIQ), and the Cohen-Hoberman Inventory of Physical Symptoms (CHIPS).

The researchers measuring stress in relation to *pranayama* selected the PSS. A frequently used psychological instrument to gauge various perceptions of stress, PSS scores thoughts and feelings to measure the "degree to which situations in one's life is appraised as stressful." Unlike previous methods, it takes a reverse route. Instead of focusing on stressful factors, such as financial loss, deaths of loved ones, or chronic illnesses, it focuses on how different stressful situations affect our feelings and our perception of stress. Based on the *Transactional Model of Stress and Coping* by Richard Lazarus, a psychologist and an unabashed advocate of the importance of emotion, the PSS leans more on reactions to stress than to its causes.

The triumphant course of PSS has traversed well beyond merely tabulated reactions. Its implications have included objective biological markers of stress and increased risk for disease among persons with higher perceived stress levels. For example, those with higher scores (suggestive of chronic stress) on the PSS fare worse on biological markers of aging, cortisol levels, immune markers, depression, infectious disease, wound healing, and prostate-specific antigen levels in men.

Ten basic questions are asked, and it is worthwhile to review them to have a better handle of how *pranayama* can affect stressed individuals:

1. In the last month, how often have you been upset because of something that happened unexpectedly?

2. In the last month, how often have you felt that you were unable to control the important things in your life?
3. In the last month, how often have you felt nervous and stressed?
4. In the last month, how often have you felt confident about your ability to handle your personal problems?
5. In the last month, how often have you felt that things were going your way?
6. In the last month, how often have you found that you could not cope with all the things you had to do?
7. In the last month, how often have you been able to control irritations in your life?
8. In the last month, how often have you felt you were on top of things?
9. In the last month, how often have you been angered because of things that happened that were outside of your control?
10. In the last month, how often have you felt difficulties were piling up so high that you could not overcome them?

How did Dr. Sharma and his colleagues *measure* the individual's stress?

The standard procedure was to score the ten reactions as follows:

0 = never   3 = fairly often
1 = almost never   4 = very often
2 = sometimes

The questions that invoke one's positive reactions (#4, 5, 7, and 8) are scored in the reverse order:

0 = 4   3 = 1
1 = 3   4 = 0
2 = 2

With individual scores ranging from 0 to 40, and higher scores reflecting higher perceived stress, the following results were reached:

0–13 = low stress   27–40 = high perceived stress

14–26 = moderate stress

What did these researchers find with their tool of *pranayama*?

Instant successes came with the vital parameters. A significant decrease in DBP, HR, MAP, RPP and DoP were observed in Group Two patients trained with slow pranayama. Not surprisingly, as per the science of *pranayama* discussed earlier, decreases in all these parameters represented an increase in parasympathetic and a decrease in sympathetic activities.

The most profound and persistent success came with *pranayama's* effects on stress levels, as documented through the PSS. Statistically significant reductions in PSS scores were observed in both fast and slow *pranayama* groups, compared to the control group.

Meditation Made Simple

The power of simplicity is often its ultimate strength. Endowed with an emphasis on complete freedom and free from any tutorials, it revels in unchallenged supremacy. To Shamash Aladina, this quality of simplicity seems to have come naturally. As a global teacher in mindfulness meditation based out of North London, and the bestselling author of *Mindfulness for Dummies*, he has been instrumental in infusing peace and serenity to hundreds of men and women through his art of simplistic meditation.

To the stressed out, fettered by frequent emotional and mental outbursts, Shamash's ways of meditation emerge as instantly possible, easy to grasp, and enjoyable. The experience almost verges on having fun. I loved it.

To Shamash, any posture that is comfortable to *that* individual is a good posture. You could be in the traditional lotus pose or in more unorthodox positions, such as sitting on a chair, half-reclining with support on the back, or even lying down in a supine posture.

We might think that he is loosening basic ground rules of the game and compromising the results. To the contrary, I found great rationality in these relaxations. Comfort is essentially an individual experience. A person with back pain may find the spine-straight sitting posture more congenial than the half-reclined position. Similarly, the frequently short-of-breath asthmatic patient may find the half-reclined position more soothing than lying down. An elderly person with an unstable gait would feel far more comfortable simply sitting on a chair with arms on both sides.

One cannot aspire to mental peace from a body that is restrained, rigid, and unsecure.

As for breathing, the same simple singularity is adopted—a deep but unforced inhalation, followed by an equally relaxed exhalation. A ten to twenty-minute session can start as once a day and be extended to twice a day when one becomes more in tune with the practice.

To Shamash, the concept was more important than the technique, a concept where thoughts of both past and future need to be released, again not forcibly but gently, almost lovingly. A tranquil, pleasant *present* is sought—a comforting present tense that welcomes all that is good and purposeful, despite shifting moods.

Shamash offered me a new word and I instantly lapped it up.

Kindfulness.

It was as if the word *mindfulness* had melted into the word *kindfulness.* I realized this formed the very epitome of his approach. In the pursuit of mental tranquility, a certain benevolence becomes required for the mind that may have darkened into anxiety or aggression—an attitude that endeavors to be caring—to others and to oneself. And with it comes a sense of acceptance—of who you are, where you are, and in what state of existence you find yourself. For once, I thought Shamash sounded like Reinhold Niebuhr, the American theological ethicist, who wrote in his Serenity prayer:

> "God grant me the serenity to accept the things I cannot change,
> Courage to change the things I can,
> And the wisdom to know the difference."

To Shamash, these become the attributes that need to be cultivated as one sits down to meditate. In what ways can one be mindful? Going by his approach, I was not expecting any complexities. Indeed, he keeps it very simple.

One can be mindful of one's own body with a gentle, chronological tracking of one's own framework, from toe up through the spinal cord to one's vortex. In short, this becomes a mindful sinking into the various layers of our body, system by system, organ by organ, possibly cell by cell. The same concept is applied to mindfulness breathing in the nonjudgmental following of our respiration—the entire unforced process of spontaneous inspiration and expiration.

However, mindfulness does not have to be restricted to our body process. It can be borrowed from nature. Sounds, natural and dulcet, can be allowed into and absorbed by the mind, just as thoughts or even emotions. Emotions that comfort us offer peace and solace, and are equally compatible to a mind seeking tranquility, as is the process of our quiet breathing.

A Transnational Yogi

Vasiliy Beniaminov hails from Russia. Jewish by birth, Vasiliy was young and brash when he came across a *Yogi* named Aengar, in his hometown of Kislovodsk. Two aspects of that *Yogi's* teachings attracted him instantly: the flexibility of the dictums and the universality of the goals. There was an enormous temptation to seek freedom and happiness. Vasiliy decided to pursue meditation and yoga. Years of rigorous practice and discipline followed. He traveled to virtually all corners of India, seeking from each and every one the art of meditation and yoga. A follower of *Lord Shiva*, he is now called *Siva*, while his wife, going by Hindu mythology, is named *Parvati*.

Vasiliy is currently settled in the Brighton Beach area of Brooklyn, stretching from Sheepshead Bay to Sea Gate. Presently inhabited by Russian immigrants flooding the areas after the collapse of the Soviet Union and much before by Jewish survivors of the Holocaust, this ocean-encircling landscape is riddled with shops and apartments that almost talk to each other from one's bedroom to someone else's kitchen.

I met Vasiliy there when he was 65 years old but looking 20 years younger, both in structure and demeanor. He carried the same cherubic countenance I had witnessed in Shamash from England. He lit a candle and placed it in between us as we sat on our respective mats, face to face.

His English was halted and strained. Surprisingly, though, his words and phrases of wisdom came out easily. He spoke of all of us and of everything around us as "reflections of our mind." He was emphatic about science meeting spirituality to attain "one single consciousness." He went back to the preachings of the Veda to quote the five essential elements or *pancha bhootas*: ether, air, fire, water, and earth. When aligned with Awareness, this is the avenue to achieving Oneness. Vasiliy sounded relaxed all through, harbored a gentle smile all along, and carried a refreshingly unrushed tone.

I requested him to show me some of the *asanas*. He obliged, willingly and happily, with minimal effort and with complete ease. He started with the *pranayama*, then moved on to the following sequences (see illustrations t/k):

+ *Ardha matsyendrasana*: derived from the Sanskrit *ardha*, meaning half, and *matsya*, meaning fish. A Spinal Twist Pose. The *asana* usually appears as a seated spinal twist with many variations, and is one of the 12 basic *asanas* in many systems of Hatha Yoga.
+ *Bhujangasana*: derived from the Sanskrit *bujhanga*, meaning serpent. A gentle back bend practiced from a face-down position, which warms and strengthens the spine while opening the chest.
+ *Trikonasana*: derived from the Sanskrit *trikon*, meaning triangle. Essentially a triangle pose.
+ *Halasana*: derived from the Sanskrit *hala*, meaning plow. The practitioner lies on the floor, lifts the legs, and then places them behind the head.
+ *Sirsana*: derived from the Sanskrit *sirsa*, meaning head. In the Supported Headstand, the body is completely inverted and held upright, supported by the forearms, while the crown of the head rests lightly on the floor.
+ *Matsyasana*: derived from the Sanskrit *matsya*, meaning fish, a reclining back-bending *asana*.

Vasiliy ended with the final pose of deep restoration after any yoga session—*Shavasana*—derived from the Sanskrit *shava*, meaning corpse. Essentially a Corpse Pose, where one lies down fully conscious and awake, yet completely relaxed.

Vasiliy practices meditation and yoga daily. He runs the boardwalk every morning and holds lectures and workshops that draw men and women from all walks of life.

"I don't remember being stressed out in my last thirty years," he said. "I am in good health. In fact, I have not been to a doctor for twenty years."

He then looked up to me, his mischievous eyes settling on mine. "But then, I know I should."

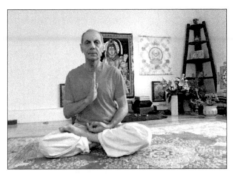

Vasiliy Beniaminov in Padmasana with Namaste pose.

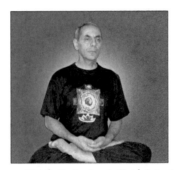

Russian yogi Vaisiliy Beniaminov in Simple Lotus position.

6

MUSIC, VIRTUAL REALITY, AND SIMPLY A TOUCH

The past which is not recoverable in any other way
is embedded, as if in amber, in the music, and
people can regain a sense of identity . . .

—Oliver Sacks

December nights are cold in New Jersey. More than a decade back, I was pursuing my residency at Raritan Bay Medical Center. As a senior resident, I was in charge of all Intensive Care Unit (ICU) admissions. Hospital nights are a different world, ruled by silent, hushed corridors. Groans, moans, and even labored breathing emerge from the darkness. The day-long overhead pages, such as "Code Blue," "Code Sepsis," and "Code Stroke," somehow dwindle in frequency. When they do occur, they scream out of a vacuum with no space for discussion. Time is tackled by the hour. Treatment is swift, objective, and decisive. Patient care becomes personal. Nurses and doctors bond fiercely.

I got a page one night to see a Gloria Sanchez in ICU Bed 5. I did not know her personally. The nurse reported that she had been having labored breathing since the evening. Despite putting her on a V mask, she had not been optimally saturating. Suffering full-blown AIDS, Gloria was riddled with multiple, opportunistic infections. In those days, AIDS medications were just beginning to take shape. People still succumbed to the wrath of this disease. Not wanting to involve my two junior residents assigned for the night before making a firm decision, I went upstairs to ICU by myself.

Gloria was in a semi-coma. A quick look and I thought I had the cause. Gloria's breathing problem did not stem from any respiratory issues, but from a growing ascites (a fluid-filled belly, usually, but not always, secondary to a liver dysfunction). Liver failure was probably causing her semi-coma state.

Nonetheless, I had little option but to relieve the ascites, and I instructed my ICU nurse to prepare the kit for paracentesis, the procedure to remove fluid from the abdomen. We had little chance to obtain Gloria's written permission, as her state of mind was beyond any decision-making capability. Besides, I considered it an emergency procedure.

As I suited up, I kept my cell phone on a corner shelf attached to Gloria's room. I marked the right flank of her abdomen as my point of entry. Gloria had her V mask in place; her eyes were closed, and her breathing was heavy. She flinched a little but remained unresponsive when a nurse in a reasonably raised voice informed her about our procedure. I was about to insert the trocar when, to my horror, I heard my phone scream out. In the ongoing rush, I had not remembered to switch it off. I watched it helplessly as it rang, and was about to ask my nurse to shut it off when something happened, which I barely anticipated.

That night was December 24, and in tune with the auspicious date, I had set my cell phone ringer to the timeless song, "Joy to the World."

Midway through the tune, I noticed movement from the corner of my left eye. Gloria's eyelashes fluttered. Her eyes opened just about halfway. Tired eyelids.

"Is it Christmas, Doc?" she whispered.

"Yes, Gloria, it is," I said. "Merry Christmas, Gloria."

"Merry Christmas, Doc."

The phone stopped ringing. The music died. Gloria Sanchez went back to her unresponsive state.

A Musical Mystery

One of the most fascinating case reports in medical science came in 1997 from the Department of Psychiatry and Behavioral Sciences of the University of Oklahoma Health Sciences Center. Dr. William W. Beatty and his colleagues described a patient who played the trombone and had been diagnosed with Alzheimer's about three years prior to his death from cardiac arrest. During his stay in a nursing home, the man gradually slipped into a state of complete dependency, needing assistance in all activities of daily living. Worse, he could no longer assemble his trombone by himself. But amid all the carnage of his life, his musical skills were sustained. In what could be termed an aesthetic triumph, the man could play notes, and in some glorious moments, even brief tunes, if his trombone was assembled, placed into his hands, and raised to his lips.

When he eventually died, his formalin-fixed brain was sent for microscopic examination. The brain had Alzheimer's written all over it. Very severe neuronal loss was evident in the hippocampal formation and other allied areas, along with a large number of neurofibrillary tangles and amyloid deposits.

Our trombone player goes down in history as the first reported case of Alzheimer's whose musical dexterities remained untouched, despite all other faculties shutting off in subservient obedience.

Should we be surprised? Maybe not. After all, isn't music the most cardinal form of expression? Wasn't melody present millions of years before we let out the first grunt and uttered our first syllable?

However experts choose to explain the eternal lines of Victorian poet John Keats, "Heard melodies are sweet, but those unheard are sweeter," we know for a fact that music traverses all objective expressions. Words can be formed, speeches delivered, and languages mastered, yet music remains free from all such dominions, being subjective and deeply integral.

The concept of using music as a source of healing is timeless. Literature shows its evidence from Biblical days. Aristotle described music as a force that purified emotions. Hippocrates, father of modern medicine, was said to have played music to treat his mental patients. Thirteenth-century Arab hospitals had music rooms. In fact, music existed much before its documentation in the writings of Aristotle and Plato. Music therapy has flowed from Mesopotamia, India, Egypt, Israel, and Greece, through the Middle Ages, the Renaissance, the Baroque Era, and into modern times.

Yet, in an age and time when belief prevailed over proof, these remained attractive propositions with no formal backing. Science was then more a calling than a quest.

Of all these, the usage of the word *om* (pronounced AUM) from the ancient Indian civilization seems to have transcended antiquity and was given serious consideration as a therapy for generalized well-being.

The word OM does not have an exact translation. It carries an acoustic attribute that is not circumscribed by any particular organ and reportedly beckons a certain pervasive calmness. Intriguing results came from the scientists of Sipna's College of Engineering and Technology in India, who digitized the analog waveforms of OM chanting to determine the average pitch and frequency modulation of the recorded versions.

Although rustic and lacking specific methods and materials, the experiment showed that persistent chanting of the word caused a decrease in the amplitude of frequency modulation waveforms.

Do these reflect a stabilizing effect on the brain under turmoil? It is too premature to reach any objective conclusion. A concurrent EEG (electroencephalogram), simultaneously looking into the prevalence of specific brain waves during the recording to correlate with the decrease in signal amplitude, would probably be the next logical step. There are multiple avenues to probe more deeply and fully, but the study does open the gate.

In the United States, what started off as an unsigned article, entitled "Music Physically Considered," which appeared in the *Columbian Magazine* in 1789, soon became official therapy in the 1800s in the form of a recorded intervention in an institutional setting at Blackwell's Island (now Roosevelt Island) in New York, along with the first recorded systematic experiment in music therapy—Corning's use of music to alter dream states during psychotherapy.

Call it incidental, but the tremendous emotional and physical benefits received by World War I and World War II veterans from music played by both professional and amateur musicians became an eye-opener for the medical fraternity to explore its boundless possibilities. While Willem van de Wall pioneered the use of music therapy in state-funded facilities, and authored the first music therapy text, *Music in Institutions,* E. Thayer Gaston, known as the "father of music therapy," formally institutionalized music as a formal course of medical management.

Call it a tragedy of errors or simply plain shortsightedness, but music therapy in the United States has yet to gather any worthwhile steam, despite holding a rich tradition for many years and boasting the single largest music therapy association in the world, which represents music therapists in over thirty countries around the globe. By contrast, Europe has been far more prolific in music therapy, particularly in terms of individual and group psychotherapy, to endorse emotional uplift and address intrapsychic conflicts. This is hardly surprising, considering that the concepts of psychoanalysis have been essentially a European contribution.

The Mozart Effect

One of the most visible, "talk-of-the-town" musical contributions came from the famed Mozart Effect. According to literature, Mozart's Sonata for Two Pianos in D major, K. 448, was written in strict sonata-allegro form, with three movements. Composed in the gallant style, it featured interlocking melodies and simultaneous cadences. Intriguingly, this was one of his few compositions ever written for two pianos.

The Mozart Effect all started with French researcher Dr. Alfred A. Tomatis who, as documented in his 1991 book *Pourquoi Mozart?* (*Why Mozart?*), flooded the ears of his selected patients with Mozart to presumably "retrain" that organ at different frequencies, and eventually promote healing and development of the brain. Two years later, scientists Rauscher, Shaw, and Ky, found temporary enhancement of spatial reasoning in those who listened to the Sonata, as opposed to those who underwent verbal relaxations or were given silence, only.

This set creative hearts on fire.

Lines of reasoning were effortlessly crossed, with books and articles pouring in, citing Mozart as the cure for stress, depression, and anxiety—and even more fascinating—as the source of sharper IQs.

Music columnist Alex Ross of *The New York Times* wrote, albeit in a light-hearted tone, that "researchers have determined that listening to Mozart actually makes you smarter," and how he has dethroned Beethoven as "the world's greatest composer." An over-zealous Zell Miller, erstwhile governor of Georgia, announced in January 1998 that his proposed state budget would include a whopping $105,000 annually to provide every child born in Georgia with a tape or CD of classical music.

All these efforts continued till counter meta-analysis from countless scientists started to show that the Mozart Effect is, in all likelihood, an artifact of arousal and heightened mood. Legislative bodies paid more attention to the credibility of the claims, with one German report concluding that " . . . passively listening to Mozart—or indeed any other music you enjoy—does not make you smarter. But more studies should be done to find out whether music lessons could raise your child's IQ in the long-term."

Quite like the magic of Mozart himself, interest in these indirect effects prevailed and continue to influence public life today. As reported by *The Guardian*, a German sewage treatment plant plays Mozart to break down the waste faster, with the belief that vibrations of his music can just about penetrate everything—including water, sewage, and cells.

The creative challenge seems to be in capturing the Mozart Effect. Going by the verdict of the *Journal of the Royal Society of Medicine*, Greek composer Yanni, with his composition "'Acroyali/Standing in Motion,' has done just that . . . with the same tempo, the same harmonic consonance, and the same predictability."

In a delightful twist, citing the same Mozart Effect, researchers have proposed this classical composition as a possible cure for epileptic patents. According to the British Epilepsy Organization, listening to the piano sonata improved spatial-temporal reasoning skills and reduced the number of seizures in people with epilepsy. More recently, research on South Carolina epileptic children actually found music to be a strong, viable manager of epilepsy.

Music and Research

Some of the most comprehensive research on the power of music has come from David Aldridge, Chairman of Qualitative Research in Medicine from University Witten Herdecke in Germany. Aldridge highlighted various anecdotal events to demonstrate that whereas language skills decline during cognitive deficits, receptivity to music remains until the late phases of the disease. Since the 1990s, research on music's effect on cognitive deficiencies, particularly on demented patients, has been prolific.

In 2001, twenty demented patients from the Department of Psychology at Surrey's University of London were subjected to autobiographical recall tasks, both with and without background music, in a repeated-measures design. Familiar or novel music was played, with the pieces being matched on three affective scales. Autobiographical recall was found to be better for those facilitated by music, as opposed to those who had to recall in silence.

Sometime in 2009, more significant research in the domain of autobiographical recall came from Professor Petr Janata, Associate Professor of Psychology at the University of California-Davis's Center for Mind and Brain. Not surprisingly, he targeted the same region in the brain that has been the darling of all studies concerning yoga, stress, and Alzheimer's disease: the medial prefrontal cortex (MPFC). Professor Janata demonstrated the sterling role of the MPFC as the cradle of the association between the features of the music heard and autobiographical memories and emotions. Evidence also indicated the recruitment of allied brain networks during the reliving process of music-evoked autobiographical memories (MEAMs).

In this study, thirteen UC-Davis undergraduates (eleven females and two males with an age range of eighteen to twenty-two years) listened to thirty song excerpts presented across two scanning runs of fifteen songs each, with songs lasting about thirty seconds. For each of these undergraduates, thirty stimuli were randomly selected from the Billboard Top 100 Pop and R&B charts for the years when they were between seven and nineteen years of age. Immediately after hearing the excerpts, the individuals were seated at a computer in a quiet room and instructed to complete a survey about their episodic memories of the songs they had signaled as autobiographically salient. Along with the post-scan memory test and assay of the content, each individual underwent a functional MRI to track and correlate relevant activities in the brain.

Running through the responses, Professor Janata observed strong associations between autobiographical salience and memories thick with emotions and vivid remembrances. On average, each participant recognized about seventeen of the thirty excerpts, and of these, thirteen carried moderate or strong associations with an autobiographical memory.

The fMRI images were equally fascinating. They showed that the degree of autobiographical salience had remarkable correlation and correspondence with the amount of activity in the dorsal part of the medial prefrontal cortex.

From here, an extraordinary venture followed. With a firmly held hypothesis that the MPC held music and memory together, Professor Janata and his research team actually tracked the inner trajectory of a rendition or score heard as it meandered across the twenty-four major and minor keys that are the foundation of Western tonal music.

They tracked the tonal progressions with sequential brain scans, and to their delight, the regions of the brain that retrieved memories fell along the same track of the tonal progressions. In fact, the stronger the autobiographical memory, the greater the tracking activity.

Two years later, Vinoo Alluri and his colleagues from the Finnish Center of Excellence at the University of Jyvaskyia in Finland, took a step beyond the work of Professor Janata. They dove more deeply into the subtle aspects of a musical rendition, including rhythm, tonality, and timbre, and correlated with the areas of the brain affiliated and responsible for their processing. In this logical and intuitive study, they found a wide network of brain structures to be involved and activated during music listening, including but not limited to, cognitive areas of the cerebellum, cortical, and subcortical areas.

Professor Petri Toiviainen, one of the collaborators in the research, was emphatic in his conviction and reported that, "Our results show for the first time how different musical features activate emotional, motor and creative areas of the brain. We believe that our method provides more reliable knowledge about music processing in the brain than the more conventional methods."

Why did Professor Toiviainen think theirs was a unique endeavor? Simply because this was the first time such a study was conducted using real music to replace the artificially constructed, music-like sound stimuli that had been used in past studies. To that end, participants listened to a piece of a modern Argentinian tango, while researchers analyzed the musical content of the piece, showing how its rhythmic, tonal, and timbral components evolved over time. They then compared the brain responses and the musical features.

The results were a testimony to the diversity and depth of music in its relationship to our brain. Listening to music, as shown in the study, recruits not only auditory areas of the brain, but also a wider network of areas. While the motor area of the brain processed the musical pulse, authenticating the idea that music and movement are entwined, rhythm and tonality involved the limbic area, known as an emotional hot spot.

As we realize now, the hub at the prefrontal cortex and the promises of autobiographical memory recovered by music, has become a passionate pilgrimage for researchers. Two years later, in 2013, scientists Amee Baird and Severine Samson from the University of Newcastle in Australia, focused on patients with severe acquired brain injury (ABI). Their daring goal was to prove that popular music could evoke autobiographical memories. Accordingly, five ABI patients, along with matched controls, listened to extracts from Billboard's Hot 100. The study line recalled Professor Janata's experimental approach of playing songs heard in the past. This time, however, the renditions were taken from the whole of the patients' life span, starting from the age of five, and familiarity was sought through a questionnaire, the Autobiographical Memory Interview (AMI), and neuropsychological assessment. Invariably, the songs that aroused memory buried after the brain injury were found to be more familiar and more well-liked than songs that failed to trigger a positive response.

Music and Alzheimer's:
The Tentative Approach

As recently as 2016, José Carlos Millán-Calenti, along with his colleagues from the Gerontology Research Group, Department of Medicine, at the Universidade da Coruña, in Spain, conducted a systematic review of randomized controlled trials (RCTs), focusing on the nonpharmacological management of agitation, specifically of AD patients, with the aim of making evidence-based recommendations about the use of specific intervention strategies. Of all the other nonpharmacological methods assessed, including cognitive stimulation/training, behavioral interventions, physical exercise, therapeutic touch, aromatherapy, and bright light therapy, music therapy stood out as one of the most promising and profound.

The results were particularly visible when the intervention was geared specifically for a particular individual. In other words, maximum benefit was obtained when music that categorically related to evoking positive memories *unique* to a patient was played, as opposed to any generic versions for the entire group in context. Equally strong results were obtained when music was interactive, beckoning active participation with clapping, singing, and dancing.

The researchers used a standard and popular scale to assess agitation, the BEHAVE-AD, which covers behavioral symptoms in seven categories: paranoid and delusional ideations, hallucinations, activity disturbances, aggressiveness, diurnal rhythm disturbances, affective disturbances, and anxieties and phobias (a higher score indicates more severity). The researchers probed the long-term effects of passive (listening to music from a CD player) or interactive (including clapping, singing, and dancing) music therapy, lasting for ten weeks.

A higher, long-term reduction was observed in behavioral symptoms in the interactive music group (n = 13), compared with the passive music group (n = 13) and no-music control group, which received the usual care rendered (n = 13).

The music facilitators included two music therapists, four occupational therapists, and six nurses. Each intervention was performed once a week and lasted 30 minutes. Individualized music was selected, related to specific positive memories for each participant.

The results were gratifying but not surprising, as the scores of five items of the BEHAVE-AD—paranoid and delusional ideations, activity disturbances, aggressiveness, affective disturbances, and anxieties and phobias—were significantly reduced in the group with interactive music.

How long did these positive benefits sustain? Sure enough, as this experiment showed, the effects on decreasing agitation did not last long, with benefits dwindling progressively, and eventually disappearing, after three weeks from the cessation of the interventions.

What does all this indicate? Simply that the effects are contingent on the active involvement of the patients concerned—just like, we may add, the good effects of a company-driven drug. We walk the same paths here, except in the glorious differences relating to adverse effects and tolerance—both of which are the perilous effects of a prescribed pill.

These results also revisit a fundamental concept of music therapy, or for that matter, any nonpharmacological therapy. When it comes to the treatment or management of cognitive disorders, the approach needs to be patient-centric, not the *en-masse* pillage, which pills inflict. We remind ourselves again and again that every Alzheimer's disease is different, just as every individual is unique.

Intriguingly, more than MDs, nurses have championed the use of music therapy as an indispensable intervention for patients with dementia and allied cognitive disorders. In an article published in *Clinical Nursing Research*, author H. Ragneskog, among others, described the reactions of five demented patients to three different types of music during dinner. The entire episode was filmed. One of the study's restless patients showed decreasing agitation, and the other patient actually fed himself more than usual, while in general, all patients preferred to spend more time with dinner as the music lingered.

Music as an Evidence-Based Therapy: The Muddy Trail

By this time, skeptics might start smelling a flimsy proposal on the way and issue a warrant to arrest my unfounded jargon. But I advise them not to rush into a verdict, as I also believe that in today's practice of evidence-based medicine, music, alone, cannot be considered a singular and curative therapy for any organic or inorganic disorders, especially Alzheimer's.

However, the fault lies not in music as a donor, but in *us* as recipients.

Let us take refuge in *Cochrane Collaboration*, published by John Wiley and Sons, Ltd., to get a bird's-eye view of music as a therapy for people with dementia. In this extensive and exhaustive study, authors Annemiek C. Vink and colleagues from the ArtEZ School of Music in van Essengaarde, The Netherlands, scoured major health-care databases to analyze randomized, controlled trials that reported clinically relevant outcomes of music therapy in the treatment of behavioral, social, cognitive, and emotional problems of older people with dementia.

The authors borrowed the definition of music therapy from the World Federation of Music Therapy, which defined it as "as the use of music and/or its musical elements (sound, rhythm, melody, and harmony) by a qualified music therapist, with a client or group, in a process designed to facilitate and promote communication, rela-tionships, learning, mobilization, expression, organization, and other relevant therapeutic objectives in order to meet physical, emotional, mental, social, and cognitive needs."

Accordingly, the researchers entertained two types of music therapy: receptive and active music. Predictably, receptive is all about listening to music by a therapist who sings or selects recorded music, as opposed to active music therapy, where individuals are actively involved in the act of playing music, be it instrumental, vocal, or even dance. As far as receptive therapy goes, the emphasis is on the therapist, who must be adequately trained to select and apply musical parameters that are customized to each patient's needs and goals.

The researchers looked into the outcome measures that essentially centered on any alterations in the presence of the typical behavioral problems that Alzheimer's patients presented, including wandering, verbal agitation, and general restlessness. Attention was also given to any changes and improvements in cognition, emotional well-being, and social behaviors. All behavioral and psychological tools were accepted and taken into consideration.

The research proceeded as follows, and I urge my readers to take a deep look at its methodologies, as the fallacy of the entire research analysis just might lie in the very process with which it was conducted.

In the first version of the 2003 review, researchers first identified 354 references related to music and dementia. Of these, 254 were immediately eliminated because they did not refer to a "research study" and came out as anecdotal events. A further seventy-four studies were discarded because they involved patient series or case studies. A total of twenty-six survived, of which only five received a nod of approval based on the inclusion criteria. In 2008, 18 more studies were reviewed, of which three remained active. Only two finally entered the arena from the 2010 review.

In the ten total studies that made it to the final round, both individually-based receptive music therapy interventions and active group music therapy were examined. In the first category, patients' choices were considered. Seven questions were asked across the board for all ten studies—questions that are typically addressed to any research-based study.

Did the studies use appropriate "blinding"?
Were incomplete outcome data addressed?
Were the results free of bias or selective reporting?
Did the studies involve allocation concealment? (a procedure implemented in a randomized control trial, where the individuals who screen and separate the candidates into two or more arms of a study, are blinded)

Was there adequate sequence generation? (indicating a low risk of selection bias)

Armed with these standard questions, the researchers nosedived into the individual studies to usurp both their good and bad aspects. Based on their observations, the writing on the wall was clear:

Most studies were poorly reported in terms of interventions, rationales, and chosen procedures.

Most studies paid little heed to the correct methods of randomization.

No study provided adequate information on the blinding of the care provider.

In a nutshell, all studies failed in the standard validity items shadowing the methodological qualities of most of the studies.

I will highlight one of these aforementioned studies to demonstrate why music as a therapy failed in the eyes of contemporary scientists and statisticians.

L. A. Gerdner from Health Services Research and Development, Center for Mental Healthcare and Outcomes Research, at the University of Arkansas for Medical Sciences in Little Rock, tried to show the effects of individualized versus classical "relaxation" music on the frequency of agitation in elderly persons with Alzheimer's disease and related disorders. He recruited 39 patients from six long-term care facilities in Iowa. For about six weeks, they listened to standard classical pieces from "Meditation: Classical Relaxation, Vol. 3," an anthology of classical composers, including Grieg, Beethoven, and Schubert. After a two-week wash-out (to muffle the effects of the recorded music), family members were asked through the Hartsock Music Preference Questionnaire about the preferred musical items of their related patients. Examples included Glenn Miller's "In the Digital Mood" or Perry Como's "Pure Gold."

Accordingly, these pieces of music were played for an additional six weeks. Each intervention was presented for 30 minutes, twice a week. The researchers used a repeated-measures analysis of variance with Bonferroni post-hoc (from the Latin, meaning "after this") tests, a multiple-comparison post-hoc correction used when performing many independent or dependent statistical tests at the same time. The results showed a significant reduction in agitation, during and following, individualized music, compared to classical music.

The scientists rebuffed these findings, as follows:

"The analyses described are not the correct analyses for the data. Each individual assessment for each patient was entered into the analysis, creating a file of thousands of observations, which were then analyzed, taking no account of the correlation between observations belonging to one patient. The cross-over nature of the design was ignored after a statistical test was said to show that order of treatment was not significant. Count data usually require a transformation before analysis, but there is no evidence that this was investigated.

Consequently the results cannot be accepted."

Flawless dissection. Indeed, both the analysis and crossover designs were lacking in specificity. Worse, the Bonferroni post-hoc test lacked power. It was used precisely to limit the possibility of obtaining a statistically significant result when testing multiple hypotheses. With no statistical significance achieved, the results fell flat.

No care is considered standard unless it is statistically significant. Identical verdicts were handed out to the remaining nine studies. Researchers found inadequacy in their various facets, including interventions, rationales, and chosen procedures. Blinding of the care provider, (an essential component of unbiased trials where providers are not aware of the treatment options meted out, was not found in any of the nine studies. Furthermore, analysis of the crossover trials ignored any plausible crossover designs.

These reactions hit the very belly of medical research—in terms of incorporating holistic options within the framework of standard innovations. The situation only became stickier when it approached the idea of music as therapy.

As I have hinted earlier, the problem lies in our mindset. It is useless to force down one's throat the trademark trials and tribulations to which a drug is subjected. For it is *not* a drug. It is an internal feeling, a subjective choice, a mood elevator that is at once personal and momentary. I say momentary only because the same piece of music that comes as rejuvenating, refreshing, and reviving can turn passé, dispensable, and ordinary at another time of day or in another mood of the mind. In other words, we are caught between music over mind versus mind over music. While certain music has been shown to have the capability of taming the untamed, for most individuals, receptivity of the mind takes precedence over music, per se. We go overboard trying to demonstrate the benefits of music without having the knowledge or understanding of how it actually works and achieves its outcomes.

"But it works!" Andrew DeNicola bellowed to me when I asked him about the benefits of music. Affiliated for more than thirty years with J.P. Steven High School in Edison, New Jersey, DeNicola received a nomination for a Grammy Award as a music teacher.

"How do you think music helps your students, or yourself, for that matter?" I said, as we sat in his office, while his students rehearsed.

"Very simply, it relieves the stress," he said. "I see these students. Their nerves are shot. But when they come to me, and when they play with me, they are instantly calmed. Something happens. I don't know what."

The Curious Case of Dawn Shilling

Dawn Shilling was a twenty-two-year-old patient who was admitted to our hospital in a state of complete unresponsiveness, due to a drug overdose after a fight with her boyfriend. The Glasgow Coma Scale, the standard neurological scale to assess a patient's conscious state, read 5 out of 12. Neurologists ordered an MRI of her head, which showed features suggesting anoxia encephalopathy. She remained bed-bound, on mechanical ventilation and essential comfort medicines. With no meaningful expectations, our hospital neurologist called her family members to explain the future course of action. The idea was to get her family's opinion for either continued therapy or withdrawal of active care. Accordingly, the Bioethics Committee was summoned.

It was explained in painful detail how Dawn would remain bed-ridden and tied to ventilation with little to no to chance of meaningful recovery. All family members, including her sisters and brothers, agreed to the futility of further care, all except John, Dawn's father, a retired construction worker who had bent over backwards to raise his children. After Dawn's mother died of a sudden stroke, Dawn was all John lived for, and he refused to budge, despite efforts by social workers, clinicians, and other family members. He was a religious man who reminded me more than once that, "doctors prescribe, God cures."

Active management continued, despite the administrative eyebrows that continued to rise with each passing day. I shifted Dawn to a quieter room, away from the hustle and bustle of the central nursing station. I saw no reason for meaningless weather channels and TV soap operas in her room and recommended Gospel music, much to the delight of her father, who remained steadfast day and night besides her bed, half-reclined on an armchair. I told him to talk and read scriptures to Dawn, as if she was listening, which he did in unfailing devotion.

Nothing happened, and nothing moved. We maintained the ventilation management, the peg tube feeding, the IV fluids, and the Gospel music. One day, John called me late one evening, his voice trembling.

"I think I saw Dawn's eyes roll over. And her fingers trembled. Maybe she is communicating?"

I did not have the heart to tell him that those could be natural movements, periodic and involuntary reflexes. The following morning, as I did rounds with my residents, I tried something different. I lowered my voice, and slid my ungloved index finger into Dawn's half-crumpled palm and whispered to her.

"If you can hear me, Dawn, you can squeeze my finger."

After what seemed like forever, Dawn's fingers quivered, subtle, and slight, almost in protest. I looked up at John, who stood at the other end of the bed, his lips trembling, his eyes a raging river of tears. I knew the battle was far from over. I wanted nothing to change, I wanted traditional medicine to stay back, with only gospel and John sustaining the moment.

Dawn recovered, muscle by muscle, and motion by motion. One morning, her eyes danced to my wishes. One afternoon, she consumed her first liquid diet in two months. A month later, she was wheeled out of Room 516, followed by twenty joyous family members.

Did Dawn recover naturally?

Was she an exception to the rule?

Did John's soothing words, day in and day out, unplug her clogged brain?

Did the relentless gospel music awaken her comatose brain?

We do not have answers to any one of these questions. We do know that Dawn turned around—against all medical dictates. We do know that other than ventilation management and peg tube feeding, nothing medical was done or offered. And we know that the room was flooded with music of the most profound depth and demeanor. We will do well to keep our perspectives right here.

The worst we can do is to place Dawn's personal experience among other coma patients, play the gospel music, and search for statistical significance.

We over-glorify facts and figures while the magic of personal healing gets demonized as exceptional and coincidental. More objectively, music becomes that unseen bridge, across which memories, dead and defunct, become recollections, viable and visible.

I will end this discussion on music as therapy and healer with Oliver Sacks, one of the rare neurologists who did not let knowledge muffle the intuitive insight that can traverse the obvious. In his descriptions of his experiences with Parkinson's patients, both personal and poignant, he highlighted the absolute importance of music as a healing companion.

Several examples come out of Sacks' endless experiences: a woman with advanced Alzheimer's who was still able to memorize intricate and newly learned piano compositions; a musician grounded with Alzheimer's who could actually play and record at a higher level than before, and an elderly gentleman who knew baritone parts to *a capella* songs from memory but could not otherwise say who he was.

Dr. Sacks echoed the essences of previous experiments—that familiar and comforting music is more likely to evoke lost memories of a demented individual. He went a step further and recommended "movement" in group therapy. According to him, dance, because it is multi-modal, becomes an effective tool for infusing animation in patients who are sunk in the doldrums. Even drum circles as a possible therapy carry promise because they call upon "very fundamental, subcortical levels of the brain."

Along with all my colleagues, I cannot in any rational view call music a cure for Alzheimer's. It is irrational to believe that it will untangle the amyloid plugs. Yet, a profound truth remains—that music moves every soul. Sometimes it simmers, and sometimes it stirs. It is there, though, always in the vast and deep reservoir of our minds. It is so ingrained that it cannot be forgotten. As a temporary measure, eternal for that moment, it will remain a priceless tool of management, for both the sufferer and the caregiver. To sufferers, it offers a timeless moment to recover lost selves. To caregivers, it opens a rare window to watch their loved ones return

Virtual Reality

Andrea kept the nurses on their toes. Admitted with Alzheimer's-type dementia, with frequent displays of emotional outbursts, ranging from agitation to incessant crying spells, Andrea was becoming impossible to be handled by her brother, five years her senior. She was obviously not compliant with her medications. Although she had recovered most of her motor strength from a stroke three years earlier, her disturbed personality had not recovered. Since then, she also undergone a hemi-craniotomy to remove a brain tumor.

Andrea threw a fit at everything offered to her, and in between displayed a smile that seemed more of a neurological aberration than a symbol of happiness.

Psychiatrists did their part, but Andrea reveled in her negativity, refusing to take any medication, any vitamins, or any nutritional supplements.

"Would you like to have your food?" said one of the nurses, pleading with Andrea.

"No!"

"You did not take your blood pressure medications, Andrea. You need to take them."

"Hell, no!"

I was called more for emergency than a routine visit. Andrea had been given Haloperidol by the psychiatrist to curb her hostility, but to no avail. She would dash off to sleep, but the moment Haloperidol's effect would wane, she returned to her negativities, reverting to her trademark "No!" echoing through the corridors.

While entering her room, my nurse whispered to me.

"During surgery, I am sure the surgeon must have removed her 'yes' center. Good lord, she says 'no' to everything."

Andrea looked at me with frosty eyes. From her unkempt appearance, it was evident she was under a perennial storm. Her gown was half-open, her hair disheveled, and her parched lips twisted sideways. She looked every bit like a hostage in restraints. I smiled back. She did not return the pleasantry. I completely bypassed the usual formalities. I found it fruitless to inquire how she was doing, and instead asked softly, "Sweetheart, would you like to go home?"

She whispered back instantly.

"Yes!"

"How on earth am I supposed to tackle her, now that you promised her home?" my nurse said, fully exasperated. "You are not discharging her home, right?"

"How about bringing home to her?" I said, before explaining the destructive effects of an adjustment disorder, how it can totally derail a personality and worsen any ailments.

We soon called up Brent, Andrea's brother. I explained Andrea's condition and requested some details of the room she had been occupying before her transfer to our facility. Brent texted me a photo of her room. An exact replica was impossible in a nursing home. Instead, we procured all the pictures that were in her room at home—pictures of her grandchildren, her only son in his graduation gown, herself when she was young, arm in arm with her husband while smiling away on a ship deck, and many others.

We moved Andrea to a different room. The sun fell on it, bright and bold. The window on the eastern side of her room commanded a majestic view of a valley, immersed in green. All her home photos were kept on the side table by her head.

As she entered her new room for the first time, she looked intently at the photos and suddenly turned back.

"Where is Debbie?" she said, referring to her granddaughter.

Before I could muster a response, my nurse responded, her emotions pouring out.

"She will be coming, Andrea. They all will be coming."

This is not virtual reality.

The example cited here was all about introducing familiarity to a mind trapped in an alien ambience. This is called Simulated Presence Therapy (SPT), and has been extended further to be called "simulated family presence therapy," based on the observation that nursing home residents who receive more visits from family members exhibit less agitation and greater life satisfaction.

It first came to our attention in 1995. Patricia Woods and Jane Ashley, both registered nurses from Massachusetts, conducted research with twenty-seven nursing home residents with dementia. They all listened to an audiotape prepared by their caregivers. The results showed a substantial reduction in behavioral problems and less manifestation of verbal aggression. The choking feeling of social isolation was lessened and refreshing increases in positive behaviors were observed, including better verbalization, smiling, and singing.

The seeds of virtual reality are sown in this very concept.

As the name suggests, walking a mind through a reality that is breathlessly close yet virtual is what virtual reality entails. What once existed as a high-tech game sensed intensely through headsets is now becoming a tool for health care professionals to address depression and dementia.

The opportunity and capability to live virtually through an experience oscillating from a sublime scene to a thrilling motion are at once rejuvenating and refreshing. Mood elevation is almost a guaranteed denouement. As Keats wrote in *Endymion*, "A thing of beauty is a joy forever." Likewise, beauty can be infused in the brain, quite like baby feeding. To the depressed or demented mind incapable of extracting beauty from a masterpiece, be it a framed piece of art or a cadenza, virtual reality is the ideal guide to joy—pristine and free of complication.

Soniya Kim, a physician in the San Francisco Bay area, has been placing headsets on depressed and demented patients and taking them on a joy ride. The results have been as mood-elevating as any evidence-based approach. She mentioned one six-foot, two-inch tall male patient, "hunched over and constantly anxious," reluctant to enter into any conversation, solo or in a group, who was actually singing and flapping his fingers when he "experienced" the trajectory of a bird in the virtual reality program. His visible transformation prompted instant tears in his wife.

Other than evoking joy and happiness, can virtual reality be used to revive lost memory?

Can Andrea's sudden recollection be reproduced in greater density through an even more vivid display of her past life? In short, can Andrea's past life be duplicated and brought back to her? This is an incredible stretch of the imagination, which is finding a serious foothold in modern science.

Nowhere is this as hotly pursued as in Australia. Like other countries, Australia has been hit hard by Alzheimer's, with more than 353,800 Australians currently inflicted with dementia, a figure that is expected to rise to 400,000 in less than five years. With no breakthrough on the horizon, experts fear that the numbers may spiral as high as 900,000 by 2050. The country's Bureau of Statistics cites Alzheimer's as the second leading cause of death, sandwiched between coronary artery disease and cerebrovascular death. As a result, the country is leaning toward management outside traditional norms.

Virtual reality is not an entirely novel avenue of treatment in the field of health care. It is being increasingly used in robotic surgery and medical personnel training as diagnostic tools, among various other uses. The breakthrough lies in its clinical application to psychiatry. Its rewarding effects concerning emotional emanation are being entertained in various countries.

In Australia, for example, Build VR, a Victoria-based company, uses virtual reality experiences in five categories of video scenarios: travel, adventure, animals, aquatic, and relaxation. All have been proven effective mood elevators. Patients do not even need headsets. Simple hand movements can cause changes in the landscapes or scenarios that can have elements, such as butterflies fluttering through flowers, a rowboat floating around a pond, or a family of ducks splashing in the water. What comes out of these, other than the expected emotional buoyancy, is an interactive experience that plays an equally vital role in challenging the subdued mind.

However, it is the potential to incite buried memories by reproducing past events that makes the virtual reality concept a fascinating seduction. Dr. Tanya Petrovich, manager for Business Development at Alzheimer's Australia Vic, is emphatically optimistic.

"The potential for it I think is huge," she says. "I do see lots of other uses for it and I do hope that particularly healthcare people use it more. You could have, potentially, in the near future, an old man connecting with his grandson and doing a trip through his hometown together. In terms of dementia, it's really about doing everything we can to bring back those memories."

We are probably quite a few years away from understanding the exact pathway of virtual reality for reviving memories lost in the cells clogged with amyloid plaques. As an immersive simulation of a three-dimensional environment, it can provoke our default mode network (the area considered active during and despite being in a waking-resting state), reportedly disrupted in Alzheimer's. But this remains open to speculation and further research, and until that occurs, we will happily take refuge in the momentary expressions of joy and remembrance.

Just That Touch

We are in the realm of "touch" now, that primeval bridge of bondage where languages, sentences, words, syllables, and even music become redundant. The palm on a palm, the hand on a shoulder, the sublime feel of a caress—all reach infinitely deep beneath the skin. Once a hand is held or a shoulder is touched, countless emotions surge forward from the sudden rush of an awakened heart.

While in conversation once with Dr. Constante Gil, the program director during my residency and a mentor who has shaped my medical journey, the topic drifted toward the importance and absolute necessity of touch. He mentioned his daughter's research on the sublime effects of touch on newborn babies. Dr. Karla Gil, a pediatrician in Florida, researched the beneficial effects of massage on preterm infants, including soft, subtle, gentle touching of babies as they rolled over in unspoken ecstasy. The results were amazing. Those preterm infants in the massage arm gained the optimal weight required for discharge much earlier than those in "sham massage" (a lighter-pressure caress that does not blanch the skin, as opposed to true massage, which provides just enough pressure to blanch the skin where it is touched.

It is of little wonder that a connection as profound as touching captures the interest of scientists. The temptation comes from other areas, too. Here is a form of treatment that costs nothing, is easily reproducible, creates no untoward reactions, and—perhaps most important—carries none of the dangers of a drug intake, namely adverse effects, resistance, and tolerance.

But what are we aiming to achieve by "touching" an Alzheimer's patient? We must remember that these hapless victims suffer from more than a loss of memory. As part of what we call the behavioral and psychological symptoms of dementia (BPSD), a patient must deal with a gamut of emotions, such as an expanding range of agitation, aberrant motor behaviors, including wandering away, irascibility, hallucinations, anxiety, depression, apathy, delusions, and sleep alterations. As strong components of the disease spectrum, any or all of these become important prognostic factors in a patient's capacity to impair functional activities, which become even more pronounced when the sufferer faces abject isolation in nursing home and allied facilities.

Several studies have demonstrated that almost all Alzheimer's patients have experienced at least one episode of these allied behavioral and psychological symptoms at some point during their illness. The Cache County Study on Memory Health and Aging, a collaborative research endeavor comprised of scientists from Utah State University, Duke University Medical Center, and Johns Hopkins, examined the genetic and environmental factors associated with the risk of Alzheimer's and other forms of dementia. One of their studies conclusively showed that 97 percent of a cohort of 408 demented patients experienced at least one behavioral or psychological symptom. As expected, the five-year prevalence was highest with depression (77 percent), followed by apathy (71 percent), and anxiety (62 percent). Various ranges of behavioral aberrations tended to club together, like wandering with sleep problems or irritability with persecutory delusions.

Touch endeavors to ameliorate these behavioral symptoms. As expected, we are not looking at generic, gentle random touches as modes of management. In fact, various supervised and guided forms of these non-pharmacological interventions have been developed. Some of these fall under emotion-oriented therapies; others are a part of the sensory stimulation interventions, including massage or tough therapy, while even more belong to functional analysis-based interventions and exercise therapy.

Two studies stand out for their potential and promise to remain firm evidence of the benefits of massage and touch.

Almost three decades ago, scientists Eaton, Mitchell-Bonair, and Friedmann evaluated the effect of gentle touching on forty-two institutionalized patients diagnosed with what was then called chronic organic brain syndrome.

An innovative and fascinating method of measure was adopted in the study: nutritional intake.

In this trial, patients were randomly assigned to experimental or control groups. Nutritional intake was evaluated for three consecutive weeks. During weeks one and three, all patients were encouraged to eat. In the treatment week, the experimental group members received gentle touches along with the verbal encouragement, and their results were equally fascinating. Food intake was significantly greater in the experimental group compared to the control group during the other two weeks. The researchers had every scientific right to proclaim that, as a simple intervention, "tactile stimulation" can be implemented for these patients as a viable adjunct to verbal encouragement.

Ruth Remington, from the University of Massachusetts, studied the effects of calming music and hand massage on demented patients. The goal was to demonstrate whether these non-pharmacological interventions had any effect in decreasing agitation, as is often found in these cohorts of patients. Four sections were created among sixty-eight patients who suffered from various types of dementia, including Alzheimer's, multi-infarct, or senile dementia. They included calming music, hand massage, simultaneous calming music and hand massage, and no intervention. Each intervention lasted ten minutes and was given once to each patient.

The treatment effect on "agitation level" was evaluated by using the standard, modified version of the Cohen-Mansfield Agitation Inventory (CMAI), administered by trained research assistants who, whenever possible, were blinded during treatment allocation.

The results clearly showed that each of the experimental interventions reduced agitation, compared to the group that received no intervention. The benefit was sustained and increased up to one hour following the interventions.

So why is touch not an accepted adjunct therapy for Alzheimer's dementia?

The *Cochrane Database of Systematic Reviews (CDSR)*, considered the leading resource of its kind in health care, scoured through a plethora of published articles on touch and demented patients. Its authors from the Cochrane Dementia and Cognitive Improvement Group, while nullifying most papers as failing to make the scientific cut, did acknowledge the potential—in a veiled way but as possibly viable.

I remain leery of these scientific tools when it comes to measuring the success of these subjective avenues of hope. More research should follow. Some will meet the criteria for validity, while others will fail as scientific evidence—just as meditation, music, and other holistic approaches do.

Until then, if holding a hand extracts the faintest smile from your beloved sunk in dementia, keep holding on for a few more minutes.

MEDICINE AND SPIRITUALITY: THE MISSING LINK

*In the beginning was the Word, and
the Word was made flesh.*

—John 3:16

John Morley had a lively childhood in Boston, Massachusetts, where he blossomed into a successful professional with a Master's in Statistics and vast experience as a field analyst. The business world was his for the taking. But he was also having his share of earthly challenges. His mother had succumbed to a spate of chronic diseases, ranging from diabetes to heart disorders. Then came Alzheimer's, which bottled his father into a new, airless world of captivity.

One day, John's father wandered away from their present location in New Jersey. In genuine, predatory fashion, the disease devoured his sense of existence as he drove aimlessly for hundreds of miles during one moonless night. When he was finally rescued, he was somewhere in New York on Long Island. Unhindered, his health deteriorated in rapid strides. He was in a rush, as if to see the light at the end of the tunnel. He soon passed away.

John Morley found himself at a desolate crossroads, with an abundance of challenges, which countless others have encountered. As a statistician, he could easily decode the predictable pieces of the puzzle. He could feel every step of his life as if he had walked that path for thousands of years.

And then came a "calling," an unanticipated pull to the other side of the moon, where amid the earthly darkness, he had a vision, infinitely more meaningful and deeper than the thin veneer that defined his earth.

Becoming Father John, he strode out to his new, searching world.

As we sat in his cozy office, I learned from Father John about his life, his philosophy, and his mission. A table lamp lit two pictures hanging on the wall behind us. One showed Jesus with His flock of sheep, and the other the smiling face of Mother Teresa. Both carried incredible nostalgia for me. The former took me to my convent school days. The latter was a personal remembrance that I treasure every second.

Father John has traveled far and wide, from Vatican City to the Holy Land. His intellect has ventured even further. From Christianity to Buddhism to simple humanism, he had let his mind follow the whole arc of his spiritual desires. He found a common thread in all these ways of life. Suddenly, he came to know his goal in life, his mission—*the path less traveled*—that he knew would make a difference. He would bring spiritual tranquility to men and women in emotional and physical distress. He would pray for them and *with* them, and together embark on a journey, however momentary, to find a land of eternal peace.

At 6'2" tall, decked in spotless black attire, with a pair of eyes almost pleading love and mercy, and a solemn smile forever hanging from his lips, Father John was as strong and as wanted as any lifesaving treatment.

"Why did you choose to be in a hospital?" I said, sensing his passion to be with distressed souls.

"What better way to serve God than through His creations?" he said gently. "Patients appeal to me much more than any administrative work of a church."

So what is Father John's job description? To my deep dismay and deeper embarrassment, I realized I had little knowledge of his insurmountable contribution to patient well-being. My tunneled views on inpatient care were stuck with intravenous and oral drugs, a plethora of lab and imaging investigations, and algebraic discussions with patients and their immediate members. My rushed assumptions had thought of Father John as someone who was beckoned into a room filled with family members in a flood of tears, standing helplessly in front of a gasping body.

I was utterly way off-track. And I was not the only one. I took an informal survey of what others felt about Father John. The answers I received were typical and a tragic reflection of how patient care is viewed and practiced in today's world:

He is a priest who needs to be on board to satisfy hospital regulations.
He prays when a patient expires.
I think he is part of a counseling program.
Does he come during a CODE BLUE?
I am not sure. Good question. So what does he exactly do?
I have no clue. But I do see him walking down the corridor once in a while.
How am I supposed to know? I don't see him in any committees or meetings.

How, then, does Father John serve our hospital?

Truth be told, if there is anyone who spends more time with patients and their dear ones than any physicians, nurses, and social workers, it has to be Father John. Not in discussions, questions, or giving verdicts. Not in standing at the foot of the bed, mouthing diagnosis and prognosis. But in interactions, intimate and soothing, seated at a patient's bedside, with compassionate hands, either folded in prayer or holding the nervous ones of others.

"Do you meditate?" I said.

"Yes, when in deep prayer."

"Does it help you?"

"Of course. You find a lot of peace. Especially during times of stress."

I was at the Critical Care Unit one busy morning for a patient with congestive heart failure. Betty Ellmers was a frail woman in her mid-80s, whose past medical history read like a medical textbook. She had most of the major diseases one can imagine, including diabetes, hypertension, and hyperlipidemia, and all their complications, including coronary artery disease, peripheral vascular disease, and stroke.

This was not the first time Betty had been institutionalized. In fact, she had been under my supervision at least three times over the past four years. For predictable reasons, her heart fails, the lungs fill up with fluids, and she presents with acute shortness of breath.

This time was no exception, except that she refused to interact. Her lips were sealed. There was no agitation, tantrum, or crying spell, just taut silence. Betty was tired—tired of the cyclical, repetitive states of her existence. She was giving up on life and refused to budge from her adopted silence. Although she quickly responded to intravenous Lasix, felt less dyspneic, and was soon out of bed in a chair, she remained nonchalant and unmoved by her progress

That morning, as I was about to enter her room, I saw Father John inside. He and Betty were seated and holding hands. They seemed to be in prayer. I stepped back to give them their privacy. When I returned to Betty's room, she was lying on her bed. I wished her good morning. She did not reply. Instead, she smiled back—a luxurious full-teeth smile that reminded me of how she had appeared five years earlier.

Seeking an Open Mind

I have always believed that science has an opportunity to expand beyond its current boundaries if it embraces the eclectic ideas of spirituality. The individualistic aptitude of science pursuing the rationality of solitary parts of our system, be it our body or the universe, would stand in brighter light if wedded with the holistic approach of examining the entirety of those very parts.

I am aware that I am treading into a battle-scarred field that has long cradled this endless feud between the upholders of objectivism and believers in subjectivism, each of whom have called the other counterproductive. Call it what you may, at the end of the day this seeker-versus-pursuer conflict is still striving for one universal verdict —the truth.

It is refreshing to see researchers who are examining the effects of meditation and yoga adopt the latest technology we have, in terms of PET scans and functional MRIs. It is equally refreshing to see more meditators stepping forward to lend their heads to probe and study.

I am leery of terminologies. Alternative, complementary, integrative, and mainstream are all medicines meant for the sufferer. An official Harvard Medical School definition of these terminologies runs as follows:

"Alternative medicine refers to those practices explicitly used for the purpose of medical intervention, health promotion, or disease prevention, which are not routinely taught at U.S medical schools nor routinely underwritten by third-party payers within the existing U.S. health care system."

Why would you call a branch of medicine "alternative" when more than 80 percent of the global population uses it to their benefit? At a fundamental level, are not all of them essentially various options to be tried for the ease of suffering?

We must insist on valid options, of course, as all of us know that there should be zero margin of error when it comes to addressing and managing human suffering. The process of validation, however, does not have to be identical. In their criticism of trials justifying holistic medicine, biostatisticians will point toward the Hawthorne Effect, a phenomenon in which experimental participants are influenced by the very knowledge that they are in a trial. They will also bring forth the fallibility of a perfect placebo in nonpharmacological trials. On top of that, the impossibility of achieving statistical significance without a double-blind study, where both participants and researchers are "blinded" and made unaware of the options, are considered genuine reasons to dismiss such trials as a sham.

The brave healing step comes right from here. It is futile to hold the notion that the same trial design meant for a drug will be valid for subjective approaches, such as meditation or music. Just as double blindness is tough to demonstrate in such subtle training exercises like meditation, drug resistance is equally impossible to capture in a six-month trial, especially when a drug can come out cleanly victorious only to stumble after years of use. These are necessary challenges that only reflect our own journey toward that truth we offer to suffering humans.

Two separate examples will drive home the issues to which I allude.

I start with Clopidogrel. If the name does not ring a bell, then Plavix should, as the brand name of this generic, antiplatelet drug. This oral compound works against platelets, inhibiting their activation and aggregation. In a society where ischemic heart disease rules the world as the biggest of all killers, Plavix appears as the bedroom Pope to all reeling under the audacity of its omnipresence.

An unconditional hats-off to those scientists who created this agent of hope and cheer. Yet, hardly a few years more than a decade have passed, and we have already witnessed creases on its forehead. This is the tragic trajectory of a celebrity drug that threatens to stop right in the middle of the tracks.

Let us take an objective look.

In 2005, Dr. Mark S. Sabatine and his entourage of colleagues and students received grant support from Bristol-Myers Squibb, Sanofi Aventis, and the national Heart, Lung, and Blood Institute for a research study that was to be termed CLARITY-TIMI 28. Decoded, this high-strung terminology came out as Clopidogrel as Adjunctive Reperfusion Therapy (CLARITY) and Thrombolysis in Myocardial Infarction (TIMI).

As the phrase suggests, this landmark trial was all about demonstrating the benefit of adding Clopidogrel to the existing treatment of myocardial infarction. Clopidogrel was already being used, combating any documented atherosclerosis (hardening of the arteries), a condition in which plaque builds up inside the arteries. This time, Dr. Sabatine and colleagues extended its benefits to patients with the most severe form of atherosclerotic coronary artery disease, the dreaded ST elevation Myocardial Elevation, as detected from an EKG.

Enrolling a staggering 3,500 patients at 319 sites from 23 countries, and extending from February 2003 through October 2004, this trial had the crimson-red flavor of a mega-trial. A perfect double blind 1:1 ratio for either Clopidrogel or placebo treatment, a statistical power based on the enormous number of participants involved, and firm primary efficacy end-points, such as re-occlusion of arteries and death or hospital discharge, made it a picture-perfect, modern-day trial.

The results were a joy to the scientific world, and a huge relief for those hearts destined to clot. With an initial, loading dose of 300 milligrams, and a daily dose of 75 milligrams, Clopidogrel resulted in a 36 percent reduction in the chances of a re-occlusion of the infarct-related artery or death or recurrent myocardial infarction—a substantial help for any massive heart attack. Plavix rolled in like the chariot of Alexander the Great, undaunted and victorious.

In 2008, sensing a red flag somewhere and somehow, Daiichi Sankyo and Eli Lilly funded a trial led by Dr. Jessica L. Mega that also included Dr. Sabatine from the previous landmark trial. More subdued than its predecessor, this research had 162 healthy subjects from six studies who were on Clopidogrel.

But before that, a red flag was unfurled from the observation that not all patients with heart attacks on Clopidogrel had the same protective response as was thought a few years back. Scientists in the lab had detected that the genes encoding the enzyme cytochrome P-450 (CYP), which are required for the necessary biotransformation of Clopidogrel to an active and effective metabolite, are actually polymorphic. A simple understanding of polymorphism in genetic science tells us that this points to having more than one allele (one of two or more alternative forms of a gene that arise by mutation), which may lead to the abnormal expression or production of an abnormal form of the gene. Anyone in the lab could smell a looming disaster.

The results were painfully palpable. As compared with noncarriers, those who carried the reduced function CYP2B6 allele showed less reduction of platelet aggregation in response to Clopidogrel. This was a clear message that just as all heart attacks do not have the same manifestations, all individuals do not show the same genetic appetite for the same drug.

A clearer message emerges—that a perfect trial may not necessarily lead to a perfect drug. Caught in the thick traffic of variable genes and changing environment, our biology is never etched in stone. Therefore, determinism—the process of simple derivations from conditions and laws—must have a democratic mindset.

Revisiting Yoga

Without further ado, we return the another piece of the spectrum to ask if there is there more to yoga than exercise. For example, can its spiritual connotation bring further benefit?

J. A. Smith and his colleagues from the University of Southern Mississippi in Hattiesburg asked these tantalizing questions in an intriguing study conducted in 2011 with eighty-one undergraduate students with mild to moderate depression, anxiety, or stress. They were assigned to one of three groups: integrated yoga (exercise integrated with an ethical/spiritual component), yoga purely as exercise, and a control group that received neither of the two.

The results were visible and pleasing to the eye. Both the integrated and yoga exercise groups showed decreased depression and stress, an increased sense of hopefulness, and increased flexibility, compared to the control group. Only the integrated yoga group experienced decreased anxiety-related symptoms. Skeptics may doubt the denouement. Their remorseless logic would point out that all these could be a placebo effect. Improvements in depression and stress without using robust diagnostic criteria would be trashed as pompous platitudes.

Statisticians can look for further statistical significance and will decry the "increased sense of hopefulness" as the sham enthusiasm of individuals who were hell-bent on bringing an ancient practice to the foreground. Indeed, this study, and those similar to it, lack the intricacies of a trial befitting a drug in question, and are almost always dismissed as suffering from rustic simplicities.

Smith possibly kept these hurdles in mind and did what he could to keep the bastions of modern medicine at bay. He measured the cortisol levels of all these individuals. This was a practical interjection, as nothing seems to fascinate the modern mind more than numbers. We physicians simply love treating numbers. While many numbers are lifesaving and etched in stone, some are totally relative and subjective, dependent on the context of the situation.

Even for a presentation as individualistic and personal as pain, we have numbered it to our discretion. Therefore, while 0 is meant to indicate no pain, 10 reflects the worst pain ever. We even draw faces for those mathematically challenged. A smiling face means no pain and a miserably grumpy one reflects the other end of the spectrum. In the process we completely overlook the individual's threshold for pain. An overly sensitive patient would immediately score an eight while a patient in a rush to get out of the hospital would hold it down to a three or four. Worse, as I have seen with my residents in training, other aspects of pain—whether acute or chronic, diffuse or localized, radiating or stationary—become inadvertently sidetracked.

Returning to our research, Smith did take refuge in numbers in a valiant effort to smother all possible rhetoric amplifications. He measured the cortisol levels of all 81 participants.

Smith and his teammates were looking for an objective reflection of a relative improvement, both in stress and anxiety, and the results were flattering for the researchers. Compared to both the control group, who did neither the physical exercise nor the spiritual component, and the yoga exercise group, those who underwent both the physical and spiritual components of the practice of yoga had a remarkable decrease in salivary cortisol levels from the beginning to the end of the study.

Smith was intelligent. He must have kept the Hawthorne Effect in mind. He chose not to test the elderly, searching for peace and likely to be biased by the promise of an ancient practice. Instead, he drew from young, robust undergraduates, free from any preemptive dogmas.

Do these trials of Plavix and spirituality prove a point? They do. In both cases, problems were addressed and amendments were attempted, and what stood out, crystal clear, was the honesty of the challenges *and* the circumvention.

Honest trials show the road to be taken. Not a narrow, dead-end type of road. But one that is open to any number of lanes offering a way in or out. The best road out leading to the truth for which we had started our journey.

Annie Carpenter, considered one of the most respected yogis in the world, airs the same tone: "Although our culture tends to shrink yoga to mean only the physical, asana element I believe that yoga truly is a shamanic path, capable of leading us through transformation on all levels. Yoga reminds us what is real, and thus who we are—the light radiating from within."

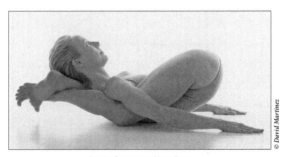

Annie Carpenter Yoga Pose.

Cure and Care

I first saw Mother Teresa when I was in sixth grade. I was returning from school one dusty late afternoon in June, an unforgiving month in Calcutta when the sun scorches the roads, even when the clock moves way past four. The bus had stopped at a red light and I noticed a group of nuns crowding around some bone-thin young boys and girls. A minivan marked, "Missionaries of Charity," stood at the corner.

"There's Mother Teresa!" someone said.

It was not hard to recognize her as I had grown up seeing and reading about her in newspapers and other media outlets.

"Hearts to love and hands to serve!" were famous words of hers for all of us.

Mother was synonymous with unconditional love and affection. An unflinching faith in God had powered her to the streets of Calcutta as she reveled in selfless service to men and women in distress. Calcutta, in turn, had opened her doors, as the city always had to anyone and everyone willing to share and care.

I saw her place her palm on the head of a young girl, whose unsure smile broke into an full grin, brimming with joy. An outpouring of tenderness followed, as Mother, not quite five feet tall and clad in a white sari with a blue border, leaned over and kissed the girl's forehead. I kept looking as long as I could, as the bus rolled away once the light turned green.

Since my childhood, I have tried to make sense of this pageantry of cure and care. I always wondered why some volunteer with fervor while others remain unmoved and indifferent. Years later, as a third-year medical student, I posed this nagging question to Dhruba Maharaj, a monk who is also one of my closest friends. We were traveling together in a truck loaded with saline and dextrose bottles, to be transported to a nearby village clinic.

"What propels you to serve so relentlessly while you could have utilized your moments in the temple?" I said, trying to fathom his feverish altruistic energy.

"Why I devote myself to service? Simply because I feel God every time I do."

His entire tone had a rustic simplicity that was embarrassingly unpretentious, I had no response. It should come as no surprise that Father John—from my present hospital affiliation—shares the exact thoughts and views.

As I proceeded through the years and tears of rigorous training, I felt a growing necessity to bring cure and care together. I personally have touched hearts more deeply when I've embraced both, and I have been instantly touched in return.

My experiences at the Calcutta Rescue Clinic are worthwhile mentioning.

Like any medical graduate nearing the end of a training period, I walked a corridor of uncertainty as earthly matters took precedence above and beyond the hauteur of being a newly created MD. You either move into a clinical subspecialty, stay in your primary field, pursue private practice, or join nursing homes as a medical officer, who in an American set-up would be called a hospitalist.

I opted instead for something that had always attracted me every time I passed its venue. Calcutta Rescue Clinic functioned on the pavement of Middleton Row, a side road that broke away from Park Street, one of the most fashionable streets of Calcutta. At the far end of the street sat two banyan trees, under which two makeshift tents were pitched. Their insides were packed with medicines, syringes, and files. The tents also carried boxes of bananas, apples, and other breakfast items. Nurses and social workers huddled inside. All of this occupied three quarters of the pavement. The remaining quarter held stools where a few doctors could sit. Patients knelt on street edges while the doctors bent down to check their hearts and lungs. If they needed a chest X-ray or blood work, those would be ordered.

Treatment was meted out beginning at six in the morning, when the entire scene quickly came to look like a medical camp in a war-torn area, with hundreds of men, women, and crying babies lining up along the street. These people came from faraway villages, most sunk in abject poverty, with no access to any heath care. Some came barefoot and some wore sandals. Some suffered from leprosy or tuberculosis, while others harbored the usual quota of seasonal diseases. Patient care would continue in broad daylight for the next six to seven hours, occupying the whole of a pavement and a half of a street. Tablets were given, injections were administered, and wounds were cleansed. By four in the afternoon, the camp had been cleaned up and miraculously vanished, and the banyan trees swayed happily over a spotless pavement.

All who came for treatment were offered a gift along with whatever medication they were given. Patients were asked what was required and necessary in their daily lives. Accordingly, some received mosquito nets, bottled juices, or blankets and quilts, while some were given sandals. The options were plenty and a source of great expectation from so many hapless people in need.

I loved this approach, this ability to touch both the mind and the heart. While this hands-on, direct mode of a healing process was rustic and lacking in technological sophistication and genuine sterilization, its benefits were clear. If a society with a rickety, temporary camp can draw hundreds of barefooted, famished men, women and children every single day, then borders must be redrawn between what is appropriate and what is acceptable.

The heat and sweat notwithstanding, one of my most treasured and satisfying moments of patient practice took place under those tents, seated on sidewalk stools. All patients with leprosy and tuberculosis were diagnosed. Slick-skin tests and sputum and wound cultures were successfully conducted. Proper medications were given. No hurried assumptions were made, for even noninfectious, systemic disorders were diagnosed, referred to nearby government-run hospitals where they could be treated. Blood transfusions, stents, even renal transplants, were arranged. Follow-up and continuity of care were done to perfection. Intense and ethical patient care actually took place on a street pavement. We treated diseases. We also healed patients, as they returned to their *bustee,* recovered and happy with a gift of their choice.

Finding Our Soul

I discussed these topics and many more with Dr. Benjamin R. Doolittle during our recent American College of Physicians annual scientific conference. Doolittle occupies a unique position in today's medical field as program director at Yale Medical School. He is also a church minister, so in many ways he is reminiscent of the good old days of medicine when a doctor could be a writer, philosopher, and spiritual thinker.

Doolittle was lecturing on if—at the end of the day—we providers of cure and care had a soul. He was referring to physician burnout and if we had the coping mechanisms to handle complete mental, emotional, and physical exhaustion. He was referring to a group of people whose profession was based on others' sicknesses, which is not always the most conducive of situations, considering the nobility and sanctity of the vocation.

How do we providers cope with internal challenges? According to a national survey comprising physicians in training, venting did not work, Xanax certainly did not work, changing jobs made everything worse, and family pressures added to the woes, although being solitary did not help, either.

What worked was a change of mindset, a practice of mindfulness, and an ability to share. A perfect example is being on call on Valentine's Day. It is a day fraught with thoroughly stressful conditions, when one is forced out of roses, restaurants, and renewed pledges to the land of moans, groans, and sighs.

Here is where a change of mindsets is warranted. How about thanking the Good Lord for the opportunity to say Happy Valentine's Day to moaning, groaning, sighing patients? How about joining the families clustered in those rooms that lodge their beloved? How about replacing adversity with an opportunity for a different perspective?

We have broken our heads trying to grapple with stress. But stress itself is *neutral*. Our minds and emotions can swing the pendulum either way. While the natural tendency to gravitate to negativity tends to be the usual course, every chance exists to reverse the arc, whether through the unconditional faith that spirituality offers or through the optimism of a rational, positively wired mind.

Quite like Dr. Richard Dawson from the Wisconsin University Laboratory, Andrew Newberg from Thomas Jefferson University Hospital pursued firm experimental pathways. He came up with hard-core evidence to show how and why spirituality heightens one's ability to be both attentive and phlegmatic. He proposed that practices as ethereal and subtle as meditation can be measured. He backed his daring proposition by measuring cerebral blood flow that was found to increase during meditation in the frontal lobe and the limbic syste—areas that traditionally form the key to attention, concentration, and behavioral-emotional states.

The frontal lobe has always captivated our attention. Ongoing studies show a direct correlation between a deranged frontal lobe and uncontrolled aggression. Almost by law, individuals exhibiting agitation and hostile behavior have been shown to have low baseline activity of the frontal cortex. Neuroscience tells us that, for some unknown reasons, the frontal part of our brain exerts an inhibitory effect on the overzealous and over-emotional nature of the amygdala and the thalamus. Almost like a guardian, one part of the brain disciplines the emotional aberrations of the other.

What makes Newberg's studies even more intriguing are the

added findings (through topographical electroencephalogram or cerebral metabolism studies), which show the activation of the temporal lobe during religious practices. The anatomical truth—that the medial temporal lobe comprises the limbic system controlling our emotions and the hippocampus is vital for memory function—formally establishes the synergistic effects of these spiritual practices.

I asked Dr. Doolittle a direct question. "Does spirituality make you a better physician?"

"What makes a better person?" he said. "Probably what makes me a better human is a good spinach salad, a gentle jog around the block, time with family, private time in prayer and meditation, and worship in church."

Physics, as an indispensable branch of science, has crossed light years in its pursuit for answers. We have moved beyond Newtonian physics into quantum mechanics to explore areas of matter energy duality. It has dared to address consciousness, rationalizing ancient concepts of a state that is neither material nor static. It is beyond a mere computable algorithm of a derivative process. In giddy delight, we learn from scientists that microtubules—those vital cytoskeletal elements and principal targets of Alzheimer's—are actually the primordial seats of our consciousness, huddled as quantum vibrations.

Dr. Everett Koop, former Surgeon General of the United States, very aptly quoted President Ronald Reagan, who once made a memorable remark while referring to his foreign policy approach.

"Trust but verify!"

This verification of trust is siphoning alternative medicine into mainstream patient care by blurring the borders and dissolving the frictions. Pharmaceutical drugs will continue to cure systems. Holistic measures will continue to reach the whole. The two together could heal the sufferer.

The Treasure of Prevention

"Prevention is better than cure," said Desiderius Erasmus. Allow me to take the next step, bend the Dutch philosopher's quote, and re-write it as follows:

Prevention is the mother of all cure.

Allow me to take you back to way before the fatherhood of Hippocrates, before any medical pedigree was created, to days of patient care when resources were scarce and ideas quite stilted, when diseases flourished and death wooed at will.

How did the "doctors" address suffering in those days?

How much was prevention, and how much was treatment?

It is amazing how many scholarly, emotional, and financial resources we have delivered since then and continue to deliver in the cure of human suffering. Yet how little do we invest in understanding the birth and development of a brewing disease before its obvious visibility.

We doff our hats to the incredible discoveries pouring in from all corners of science. In cancer, for example, since the advent of nitrogen mustard (one of the first anti-cancer drugs), through the numerous permutations and combinations of chemotherapeutic drugs, radiation, and radioimmunotherapy, to the present surplus market of monoclonal antibodies—we have been hurling anything and everything at cancer that is at our disposal. Despite all these remarkable innovative strides, patients continue to succumb to the disease.

If you dig in the mud, you will know the reason. All these drugs and procedures are truly lifesaving, except that when patients present with signs and symptoms of cancer, the disease has already traversed many miles. It is common knowledge that at this advanced stage, any malignancy is meant to be recalcitrant, not by choice, but by definition. Once the blood or lymph nodes or the nerves pick up the mutated process from the primary organ affected, we are looking at a potential disaster. Reins at this moment will fail to harness the beast, which has been let loose and is determined to kill.

The problem lies in our approach. We scientists are hunting for a light that is actually hunting for us. We are grappling with the trunk of a tree, when the roots are being left untouched. Let me give you an example.

As learned not too many years ago, research from Johns Hopkins investigators revealed that it takes nearly twenty years for full-blown pancreatic cancer to develop. According to Bert Vogelstein, MD, professor and director of the Ludwig Center for Cancer Genetics and Therapeutics at the Johns Hopkins Kimmel Cancer Center, and an investigator at the Howard Hughes Medical Institute, "many pancreatic cancer cases have a long lag time before they are detected through conventional tests. This leaves room to develop new early, diagnostic tools and intervene with potentially curative surgery."

Published in the October 28, 2010, issue of the journal *Nature*, researchers have found that it takes at least a decade for the first cancer-causing mutation occurring in a cell in a pancreatic lesion to turn into a matured cancer cell. At this juncture, if apprehended successfully, this "high-grade" lesion can very well be removed, quite like colonic polyps are removed once detected by a colonoscopy.

Subsequent to the primary mutation, it takes approximately another seven years for that cell to turn into the billions that eventually make up a plum-size cancerous tumor. At this stage, at least one of the cells in the tumor will carry the potential and ability to spread to other organs.

In this context, comparison is cruel. The body gives us as many as twenty years to detect full-blown pancreatic cancer, and yet when visible and ready to metastasize, it takes less than three years to reduce it to ashes. The literature is clear on pancreatic cancer: Patients die an average of two and a half years after metastasis.

According to Christine Iacobuzio-Donahue, Associate Professor of Pathology and Oncology at Johns Hopkins Sol Goldman Pancreatic Cancer Research Center, "so there is potentially a very broad window for screening." However, as she added, "pretty much everybody is diagnosed after that window has closed."

This is an agonizing state of affairs, where all of science seems to cluster after the disease is felt or seen, and yet turns mute when the disease process is at its slender self. This can be applied to many other branches of medical specialties.

I was in the physicians' lounge recently and saw an interesting poster by a window, titled "Hand Washing Saves Lives." It consisted of six pictures, some depicting how to wash hands, some showing tables and graphs of hard-core facts and numbers. A paper lay in front, asking physicians to sign a pledge to support this ancient, ageless, live-saving practice. There were only six signatures.

Way back in the mid-nineteenth century, the pharmacist A. G. Labarraque provided the first suggestion that hand decontamination can significantly reduce incidences of puerperal fever and maternal mortality. Not many years later, I. Semmelweis, working at the Great Hospital in Vienna in the 1840s, instituted a policy of hand washing with chlorinated lime for those leaving the autopsy room. Even in those days, the results of no formal antibiotic usage were tremendous, with a tenfold drop in the rate of maternal deaths.

History has continued to remind us of the dangers of not washing our hands. Staphylococcal epidemics in the 1950s have conclusively shown that direct contact was the main mode of bacteria transmission in nurseries.

Worse news, however, comes from Centers for Disease Control and Prevention (CDC). According to its official announcement, "On average, healthcare providers clean their hands less than half of the times they should. On any given day, about one in twenty-five hospital patients has at least one healthcare-associated infection."

All this is occurring, despite living in an era when extended-spectrum antibiotics are continuously tailored to overcome rampaging, resistant bacteria. This serves as a scathing reminder that unless we travel back to the treasures of basic practices of prevention, the roots of our suffering will not end.

What Now?

When it comes to healing Alzheimer's disease, we face an identical crisis. Can scientists detect a pathology at its very inception? Can they diagnose the disease when only a hint exists? Along with our intellectual aggression to develop new cures, we must foster an equivalent fervor to capture the disease before it can mature. In order to do that, we need to remove the rust that has collected in the arts of diagnosis that used to be considered masterpieces. We need to start all over again, as students of truth, with the belief that permanence of any solution lies in the prevention of that very problem.

Meditation and yoga, as well as spirituality and other holistic approaches offer the promise of such permanence in the art of their practice. They brew well before organs mature, and linger long after they wither. They become priceless accompaniments in our striving for a disease-free sojourn through life.

REFERENCES

AD2000 Collaborative Group, Bentham P, Gray R, et al. Aspirin in Alzheimer's disease (AD2000): A randomised open-label trial. Lancet Neurol. 2008; 7:41.

Adiswarananda S. *Meditation and its practices: A definitive guide to techniques and traditions of meditation in yoga and Vedanta.* Woodstock, VT: Sky Light Paths Publishing; 2003.

Agid Y, Buzsáki G, Diamond DM, Frackowiak R, Giedd J, Girault J-A, Grace A, Lambert JJ, Manji H, Mayberg H, Popoli M, Prochiantz A, Richter-Levin G, Somogyi P, Spedding M, Svenningsson P, Weinberger D. How can drug discovery for psychiatric disorders be improved? *Nature Reviews Drug Discovery.* 2007 Mar; 6, 189–201.

Aisen PS, Schafer KA, Grundman M, et al. Effects of rofecoxib or naproxen vs placebo on Alzheimer disease progression: A randomized controlled trial. *JAMA.* 2003; 289: 2819–26.

Albers MW, Tabert MH, Devanand DP. Olfactory dysfunction as a predictor of neurodegenerative disease. *Curr Neurol Neurosci Rep.* 2006; 6(5):379–86.

Aldridge D, Gustorff D, Hannich H-J. Where am I? Music therapy applied to coma patients. *J Royal Society of Med.* 1990; 83(6): 345–6.

Aldridge D, Gustorff D, Neugebauer L. A pilot study of music therapy in the treatment of children with developmental delay. *Complementary Therapies in Medicine.* 1995; 3: 197–205.

Aldridge D. Alzheimer's disease: Rhythm, timing and music as therapy. *Biomedicine and Pharmacotherapy.* 1994; 48(7): 275–328.

Aldridge D. Music and Alzheimer's' disease—assessment and therapy: A discussion paper. *J Royal Society of Med.* 1993a; 86:93–95.

Aldridge D. *Music therapy in dementia care.* London: Jessica Kingsley; 2000.

Aldridge D. *Music therapy research and practice in medicine. From out of the silence.* London: Jessica Kingsley; 1996a.

Aldridge D. Music therapy research: I. A review of the medical research literature within a general context of music therapy research. Special Issue: Research in the creative arts therapies. *Arts in Psychotherapy*. 1993b; 20(1): 11–35.

Aldridge D. Music, communication and medicine: Discussion paper. *J Royal Society of Med*. 1989; 82(12): 743–46.

Alladi S, Xuereb J, Bak T, et al. Focal cortical presentations of Alzheimer's disease. *Brain*. 2007; 130: 26–36.

Allen NB, Blashki G, Chambers R, Ciechomski L, Gullone E, Hassed C, et al. Mindfulness-based psychotherapies: A review of conceptual foundations, empirical evidence and practical considerations. *Aust N Z J Psychiatry*. 2006; 40(4): 285–94.

Alluri V, Toiviainen P, Jääskeläinen IP, Glerean E, Sams M, Brattico E. Large-sclae brain networks emerge from dynamic processing of musical timbre, key and rhythm. *NeuroImage*. 2012 Feb 15; 59(4): 3677–89.

Alzheimer's Association. 2016 Alzheimer's disease facts and figures. *Alzheimer's Dement*. 2016 April; 12(4): 459–509.

American Psychiatric Association. *Diagnostic and statistical manual of mental disorders (DSM-5)*. 5th ed. Arlington, VA: American Psychiatric Association; 2013.

American Psychological Association. *Diagnostic and statistical manual of mental disorders (DSM-IV-TR)*. 4th ed. (text revision). Washington, DC: American Psychological Association; 1994.

Amihai I, Kozhevnikov M. The influence of Buddhist meditation traditions on the autonomic system and attention. *BioMed Res Intl*. 2015; 2015: ID 731579.

Aminov RI. The role of antibiotics and antibiotic resistance in nature. *Environ Microbiol*. December 2009; 11(12): 2970–88.

Andersen K, Launer LJ, Ott A, et al. Do nonsteroidal anti-inflammatory drugs decrease the risk for Alzheimer's disease? The Rotterdam study. *Neurology*. 1995; 45: 1441–45.

Anderson JW, Liu C, Kryscio RJ. Blood pressure response to transcendental meditation: A meta-analysis. *Am J Hypertens*. March 2008; 21(3): 310–6.

Astin, J. Stress reduction through mindfulness meditation: Effects on psychological symptomatology, sense of control, and spiritual experiences. *Psychotherapy and Psychosomatics,* 1997; 66: 97–106.

Attems J, Jellinger KA. Olfactory tau pathology in Alzheimer disease and mild cognitive impairment. *Clin Neuropathol*. 2006; 25(6): 265–71. [PubMed]

Attems J, Walker L, Jellinger KA. Olfaction and aging: A mini-review. *Gerontology*. 2015; 61(6): 485–90.

Baddeley AD, Hitch G. Recency re-examined. In S. Dornic, ed. *Attention and Performance: 6th Symposium Proceedings*. New York, NY: John Wiley & Sons; 1977: 647–67.

Baddeley AD, Hitch GJ. (1974). Working memory. In: Bower, GA. ed. *Recent advances in learning and motivation*. New York, NY: Academic Press: 47–89.

Baddeley AD, Hitch GJ. The recency effect: Implicit learning with explicit retrieval? *Mem Cognit*. 1993; 21, 146–55.

Baddeley AD, Kopelman MD, Wilson BA. *The handbook of memory disorders*. 2nd ed. Chichester: Wiley; 2002a.

Baddeley AD, Vargha-Khadem F, Mishkin M. (2001). Preserved recognition in a case of developmental amnesia: implications for the acquisition of semantic memory. *J. Cogn. Neuroscience.* 2001; 13(3): 357–69.

Baddeley AD, Wilson B. (1988). Frontal amnesia and the dysexecutive syndrome. *Brain and Cognition.* 1988; 7: 212–30.

Baddeley AD, Wilson BA. (2002). Prose recall and amnesia: Implications for the structure of working memory. *Neuropsychologia.* 2002; 40: 1737–43.

Bahar-Fuchs A, Chételat G, Villemagne VL, Moss S, Pike K, Masters CL, Rowe C, Savage G. Olfactory deficits and amyloid-β burden in Alzheimer's disease, mild cognitive impairment, and healthy aging: A PiB PET study. *J Alzheimers Dis.* 2010; 22(4): 1081–7. doi:3233/JAD–2010–100696

Bahar-Fuchs A, Moss S, Rowe C, Savage G. Olfactory performance in AD, aMCI, and healthy ageing: A unirhinal approach. *Chem Senses.* 2010; 35: 855–62.

Baird A, Samson S. Music evoked autobiographical memory after severe acquired brain injury: Preliminary findings from a case series. *Neuropsychological Rehab.* 2014; 24(1): 125–43. doi:10.1080/096 02011.2013.858642. Epub. 2013 Nov 21.

Balasa M, Gelpi E, Antonell A, et al. Clinical features and APOE genotype of pathologically proven early-onset Alzheimer disease. *Neurology.* 2011; 76: 1720–5.

Ballard C, Gauthier S, Corbett A, et al. Alzheimer's disease. *Lancet.* 2011; 377: 1019–31.

Balsis S, Carpenter BD, Storandt M. Personality change precedes clinical diagnosis of dementia of the Alzheimer type. *J Gerontol B Psychol Sci Soc Sci.* March 2005; 60(2): P98–P101.

Ban T. The role of serendipity in drug discovery. *Dialogues Clin Neurosci.* 2006 Sep; 8(3): 335–44.

Banaji MR, Crowder RG. (1989). The bankruptcy of everyday memory. *Amer. Psych.* 1989; 44: 1185–93.

Bargh JA, Chartrand, TL. The unbearable automaticity of being. *Amer. Psych.* 1999; 54: 462–79.

Bargh JA, Williams LE. The nonconscious regulation of emotion. In: Gross JJ. ed. *Handbook of emotion regulation.* New York, NY: Guilford; 2007; 429–45.

Barnby JM, Bailey NW, Chambers R, Fitzgerald PB. How similar are the changes in neural activity resulting from mindfulness practice in contrast to spiritual practice? *Conscious Cogn.* November 2015; 36: 219–32. Epub 2015 Jul 11.

Barrett AM, Eslinger PJ, Ballentine NH, Heilman KM. Unawareness of cognitive deficit (cognitive anosognosia) in probable AD and control subjects. *Neurology.* 2005; 64: 693–9.

Bausell RB. *Snake oil science.* New York, NY: Oxford University Press; 2007.

Beach TG, Kuo YM, Spiegel K, et al. The cholinergic deficit coincides with Abeta deposition at the earliest histopathologic stages of Alzheimer disease. *J Neuropathol Exp Neurol.* 2000; 59(4): 308–13. [PubMed]

Beatty WW, Brumback RA, Vonsattel J-PG. Proven Alzheimer disease in a patient with dementia who retained musical skill in life. *Arch Neurol.* 1997; 54(12): 1448. doi:10.1001/archneur.1997 .00550230008002

Bell MA, Wolfe CD. Emotion and cognition: An intricately bound developmental process. *Child Dev.* 2004; 75(2): 366–70.

Benini A. Consciousness and self-consciousness as biological phenomena. *Schweiz Rundsch Med Prax.* 1994 Feb; 83(8): 204–9.

Bennett DA, Wilson RS, Schneider JA, et al. Natural history of mild cognitive impairment in older persons. *Neurology* 2002; 59: 198–205.

Berger A, Kofman O, Livneh U, Henik A. Multidisciplinary perspectives on attention and the development of self-regulation. *Prog. Neurobiol.* 2007; 82(5): 256–86.

Berk L, van Boxtel M, van Os J. Can mindfulness-based interventions influence cognitive functioning in older adults? A review and considerations for future research. *Aging & Mental Health.* 2016 May, 1–8. http://dx.doi:org/10.1080/13607863.2016.1247423

Berking M, Wupperman P, Reichardt A, Pejic T, Dippel A, Znoj H. Emotion regulation skills as a treatment target in psychotherapy. *Behav. Res. Therapy.* 2008; 46(11): 1230–7.

Betts J, Gullone E, Allen JS. (2009). An examination of emotion regulation, temperament and parenting as potential predictors of adolescent depression risk status. *Brit. J. Dev. Psych.* 2009; 27: 473–85.

Birks J, Flicker L. Selegiline for Alzheimer's disease. *Cochrane Database Syst Rev.* 2000; CD000442.

Birks J, Grimley Evans J. Ginkgo biloba for cognitive impairment and dementia. *Cochrane Database Syst Rev.* 2007; CD003120.

Bischkopf J, Busse A, Angermeyer MC. Mild cognitive impairment—A review of prevalence, incidence and outcome according to current approaches. *Acta Psychiatr Scand.* 2002; 106: 403–14.

Bishop SR, Lau M, Shapiro S, Carlson L, Anderson ND, Carmody J, Segal ZV, Abbey S, Speca M, Velting D, Devins G. Mindfulness: A proposed operational definition. *Clin Psychol: Sci Pract.* 2004 Autumn; 11 (3): Health Module 230.

Bishop SR. What do we really know about mindfulness-based stress reduction? *Psychosomatic Med.* 2002; 64: 71–84.

Blessed G, Tomlinson BE, Roth M., Blessed-Roth Dementia Scale (DS). *Psychopharmacol Bull.* 1988; 24(4): 705–8.

Boake C. Edouard Claparède and the auditory verbal learning test. *J Clin Exp Neuropsychol.* 2000; 22(2): 286–92.

Bodhi B. What does mindfulness really mean? A canonical perspective. *Contemporary Buddhism.* 2011 May; 12(1): 19–39.

Bokde AL, Pietrini P, Ibáñez V, et al. The effect of brain atrophy on cerebral hypometabolism in the visual variant of Alzheimer disease. *Arch Neurol.* 2001; 58:480–6.

Botvinick MM, Braver TS, Barch DM, Carter CS, Cohen JD, Conflict monitoring and cognitive control. *Psychol Rev.* 2001; 108(3): 624–52.

Braak H, Braak E. Frequency of stages of Alzheimer-related lesions in different age categories. *Neurobiol Aging.* 1997; 18: 351–7.

Braak H, Braak E. Neuropathological stageing of Alzheimer-related changes. *Acta Neuropathol.* 1991; 82(4): 239–59.

Brefczynski-Lewis JA, Lutz A, Schaefer HS, Levinson DB, Davidson RJ. Neural correlates of attentional expertise in long-term meditation practitioners. *Proc Natl Acad Sci U S A.* 2007 Aug; 104(27): 11483–8.

Britta KH, Carmody J, Vangel M, Congleton C, Yerramsetti SM, Gard T, Lazar SW. Mindfulness practice leads to increases in regional brain gray matter density. *Psychiatry Res: Neuroimaging.* 2011 Jan; 191(1): 36–43.

Brown BM, Rainey-Smith SR, Villemagne VL, et al. The relationship between sleep quality and brain amyloid burden. *Sleep*. 2016; 39: 1063–8.

Brown KW, Creswell JD, Ryan EM. *Handbook of mindfulness: Theory, research, and practice*. New York, NY Guilford Press; 2015.

Brown KW, Ryan RM, Creswell JD, Niemiec CP. Beyond me: Mindful responses to social threat. In: Wayment HA, Bauer JJ. eds. *Transcending self-interest: Psychological explorations of the quiet ego*. Washington, DC: American Psychological Association; 2008: 75–84.

Brown KW, Ryan RM, Creswell JD. Mindfulness: Theoretical foundations and evidence for its salutary effects. *Psych Inquiry*. 2007; 18: 211–37.

Brown KW, Ryan RM. Perils and promise in defining and measuring mindfulness: Observations from experience. *Clin Psych: Science and Practice*. 2004; 11(3): 242–8.

Brown RP, Gerbarg PL. Sudarshan Kriya Yogic breathing in the treatment of stress, anxiety, and depression. Part II—clinical applications and guidelines. *J Altern Complement Med*. 2005 Aug; 11(4): 711–7.

Brown RP, Gerbarg PL. Yoga breathing, medication, and longevity. *Ann N Y Acad Sci*. 2009 Aug; 1172: 54–62S.

Brunnhuber S, Michalsen A. Psychosomatik und Mind-Body-Medizin: Integrative, komplementäre oder alternative Disziplinen? Ein entwicklungslogisches Argument. *Forschende Komplementär-medizin/Res Complem Med*. 2012; 19(2): 86.

Burke MA. *Effects of music therapy on elderly extended care inpatients receiving radiation or physical therapy*. Durham, NC: Center for the Study of Aging and Human Development, Duke University Medical Center, Extended Care and Rehabilitation Center; 1995.

Burke WJ, Roccaforte WH, Wengel SP, et al. L-deprenyl in the treatment of mild dementia of the Alzheimer type: Results of a 15-month trial. *J Am Geriatr Soc*. 1993; 41: 1219–225.

Bush G, Luu P, Posner MI. Cognitive and emotional influences in anterior cingulate cortex. *Trends Cogn Sci*. 2000; 4(6): 215–22.

Busse A, Hensel A, Gühne U, et al. Mild cognitive impairment: Long-term course of four clinical subtypes. *Neurology*. 2006; 67: 2176–85.

Cabeza R, Prince SE, Daselaar SM, Greenberg DL, Budde M, Dolcos F, LaBar KS, Rubin DC. Brain activity during episodic retrieval of autobiographical and laboratory events: An fMRI study using a novel photo paradigm. *J Cogn Neurosci*. 2004; 16: 1583–94. [PubMed]

Callejas A, Lupianez J, Tudela P. The three attentional networks: On their independence and interactions. *Brain Cogn*. 2004; 54: 225–7.

Canineu LF, Paulo R, de Souza LC, Forlenza OV. Neuropsychiatric symptoms in the prodromal stages of dementia. *Current Opinion in Psychiatry*. 2014 May; 27(3): 230–5.

Carlson LE, Speca M, Patel KD, Goodey E. Mindfulness-based stress reduction in relation to quality of life, mood, symptoms of stress, and immune parameters in breast and prostate cancer outpatients. Psychoneuroendocrinology. 2004 May; 29(4): 448–74.

Carlson LE, Speca M, Patel KD, Goodey E. Mindfulness-based stress reduction in relation to quality of life, mood, symptoms of stress and levels of cortisol, dehydroepiandrosterone sulfate (DHEAS) and melatonin in breast and prostate cancer outpatients. *Psychosom Med*. 2003 Jul-Aug; 65(4): 571–81.

Carmody J, Baer RA. Relationships between mindfulness practice and levels of mindfulness, medical and psychological symptoms and well-being in a mindfulness-based stress reduction program. *J Behav Med*. 2008 Feb; 31(1): 23–33. Epub 2007 Sep 25.

Carni E. Issues of hope and faith in the cancer patient. *J Relig Health*. 1988 Dec; 27(4): 285–90.

Carter CS, Botvinick MM, Cohen JD. The contribution of the anterior cingulate cortex to executive processes in cognition. *Rev. Neurosci*. 1999; 10(1): 49–57.

Carter OL, Presti DE, Callistemon C, Ungerer Y, Liu GB, Pettigrew JD. Meditation alters perceptual rivalry in Tibetan Buddhist monks. *Curr Biol*. 2005; 15: R412–R413.

Chambers R, Gullone E, Allen NB. Mindful emotion regulation: An integrative review. *Clin Psychol Rev*. 2009; 29: 560–72.

Chan D, Woollacott M. Effects of level of meditation experience on attentional focus: Is the efficiency of executive or orientation networks improved? *J Altern Complement Med*. 2007 Jul-Aug; 13(6): 651–7.

Charlson ME, Loizzo J, Moadel A, Neale M, Newman C, Olivo E, Wolf E, Peterson JC. Contemplative self-healing in women breast cancer survivors: A pilot study in underserved minority women shows improvement in quality of life and reduced stress, *BMC Complement Altern Med*. 2014; 14: 349. doi.10.1186/1472-6882-14-349

Chesia A, Serretti A. A systematic review of neurobiological and clinical features of mindfulness meditations. *Psych Med*. 2010; 40(8): 1239–52.

Chiatti C, Rimland JM, Bonfranceschi F, Masera F, Bustacchini S, Cassetta L, Lattanzio F. The UP-TECH project: An intervention to support caregivers of Alzheimer's disease patients in Italy: Preliminary findings on recruitment and caregiving burden in the baseline population. *Aging Ment Health*. 2015; 19(6): 517–25. doi: 10.1080/13607863.2014. 954526. Epub 2014 Sep 4

Chiesa A, Calati R, Serretti A. Does mindfulness training improve cognitive abilities? A systematic review of neuropsychological findings. *Clin Psychol Rev*. 2011 April; 31(3): 449–64.

Childers RC. *A dictionary of the Pāli language*. London, UK: Trübner & Co.; 1875.

Chowdhary S, Gopinath JK. Clinical hypnosis and Patanjali yoga sutras. *Indian J Psychiatry*. 2013 Jan; 55(Suppl 2): S157-64.

Chuang D-M, Manji HK. In search of the Holy Grail for the treatment of neurodegenerative disorders: Has a simple cation been overlooked? *Biol Psychiatry*. 2007 Jul 1; 62(1): 4–6.

Cohen S, Kamarck T, Mermelstein R. (1983). A global measure of perceived stress. *J Health Soc Behav*. 1983; 24: 385–96.

Cole JC, Ito D, Chen YJ, Cheng R, Bolognese J, Li-McLeod J. Impact of Alzheimer's Disease on caregiver questionnaire: Internal consistency, convergent validity, and test-retest reliability of a new measure for assessing caregiver burden. *Health Qual Life Outcomes*. 2014 Sep 4; 12: 114. doi:10.1186/212955-014-0114-3

Collins BM, Stam HJ. Freeman's transorbital lobotomy as an anomaly: A material culture examination of surgical instruments and operative spaces. *Hist Psychol*. 2015 May; 18(2): 119–31.

Connor DJ, Salmon DP, Sandy TJ, GalaskoD, Hansen LA, Thal LJ. Cognitive profiles of autopsy-confirmed Lewy body variant vs. pure Alzheimer disease. *Arch Neurol*. 1998 July; 55(7): 994–1000.

Conway MA, Pleydell-Pearce CW. The construction of autobiographical memories in the self-memory system. *Psychol Rev*. 2000; 107: 261–88. [PubMed]

Corbetta M, Shulman GL. Control of goal-directed and stimulus-driven attention in the brain. *Nat Rev Neurosci.* 2002; 3: 201–15.

Corey EJ, Roberts JD. John Clark Sheehan—September 23, 1915–March 21, 1992. Biogr Mem Natl Acad Sci. 1995; 68: 291–302.

Courtright P, Johnson S, Baumgartner MA, Jordan M, Webster JC. Dinner music: Does it affect the behavior of psychiatric inpatients? *J Psychosoc Nurs Ment Health Serv.* 1990; 28(3): 37–40.

Cousins LS. The origins of insight meditation. *The Buddhist Forum.* 1994–96; 4: 35–58.

Crick F. *The astonishing hypothesis: The scientific search for the soul.* New York, NY: Simon & Schuster; 1994.

Csikszentmihalyi M. *Finding flow: The psychology of engagement with everyday life.* New York, NY: Basic Books; 1998.

Cuddy LL, Duffin J. Music, memory, and Alzheimer's disease: Is music recognition spared in dementia, and how can it be assessed? *Med Hypotheses.* 2005; 64: 229–35. [PubMed]

Damasio AR. Time-locked multiregional retroactivation—a systems-level proposal for the neural substrates of recall and recognition. *Cognition.* 1989; 33: 25–62. [PubMed]

Daniel JE, Weiser BP, Psonis J, Liao Z, Taratula O, Fiamengo A, Wang X, Sugasawa K, Smith AB, Eckenhoff RG, Dmochowski IJ. Direct modulation of microtubule stability contributes to anthracene general anesthesia. *J Am Chem Soc.* 2013 Apr 10; 135(14): 5389–98.

Danner DD, Snowdon DA, Friesen WV. Positive emotions in early life and longevity: Findings from the nun study. *J Pers Soc Psychol.* 2001 May; 80(5): 804–13.

Danucalov MAD, et al. Yoga and compassion meditation program reduces stress in familial caregivers of Alzheimer's disease patients. *Evidence-based Complementary and Alternative Med.* 2013; 1–6.

Danysz W, Parsons CG. Glycine and N-methyl-D-aspartate receptors: Physiological significance and possible therapeutic applications. *Pharmacol Rev.* 1998; 50: 597–664.

Daubenmier J, Kristeller J, Hecht FM, Maninger N, Kuwata M, Jhaveri K, Lustig RH, Kemeny M, Karan L, Epel E. Mindfulness intervention for stress eating to reduce cortisol and abdominal fat among overweight and obese women: An exploratory randomized controlled study. *J Obes.* 2011; 651936.

Davidson RJ, Kabat-Zinn J, Schumacher J, Rosenkranz M, Muller D, Santorelli SF, et al. Alterations in brain and immune function produced by mindfulness meditation. *Psychosomatic Med.* 2003; 65, 564–70.

Davidson RJ, Lutz A. Buddha's Brain: Neuroplasticity and Meditation [In the Spotlight]. *IEEE Signal Processing Mag.* 2008; 25(1).

Davies A. *Themes in the philosophy of music.* New York, NY: Oxford University Press; 2003.

Davies J, Davies D. Origins and evolution of antibiotic resistance. *Microbiol Mol Biol Rev.* 2010 Sep; 74(3): 417–33.

Davies S. Artistic expression and the hard case of pure music. In: Kiernan M. ed. *Aesthetics and the philosophy of art.* Boston, MA: Blackwell; 2006: 179–91.

Davies S. *Musical works and performances: A philosophical exploration.* New York, NY: Oxford University Press; 2001.

Davis PB, Morris JC, Grant E. Brief screening tests versus clinical staging in senile dementia of the Alzheimer type. *J Am Geriatr Soc.* 1990 Feb; 38(2): 129–35.

Dawson DV, Welsh-Bohmer KA, Siegler IC. Premorbid personality predicts level of rated personality change in patients with Alzheimer disease. *Alzheimer Dis Assoc Disord.* 2000 Jan–Mar; 14(1): 11–9.

de Bruin EI, Formsma AR, Frijstein G, Bögels SM, Mindful2Work: Effects of combined physical exercise, yoga, and mindfulness meditations for stress relief in employees. A proof of concept study. *Mindfulness.* 2017; 8(1): 204. doi:10.1007/s12671-016-0593-x

de Zoysa P. The use of Buddhist mindfulness meditation in psychotherapy: A case report from Sri Lanka. *Transcult Psychiatry.* 2011 Nov; 48(5): 675–83.

Descartes, R. *The philosophical writings of Descartes, vol. II* (trans. Cottingham J, Stootho R, Murdoch D). Cambridge, UK: Cambridge University Press; 1984.

Devanand DP, Michaels-Marston KS, Liu X, et al. Olfactory deficits in patients with mild cognitive impairment predict Alzheimer's disease at follow-up. *Am J Psychiatry.* 2000; 157(9): 1399–1405.

Dissonance. *The American Heritage Dictionary.* 4th ed. New York, NY: Houghton Mifflin Harcourt; 2001.

Dobkin PL, Zhao Q. Increased mindfulness—The active component of the mindfulness-based stress reduction program? Complement Ther Clin Pract. 2011 Feb; 17(1): 22–7.

Doty RL, Shaman P, Applebaum SL, Giberson R, Siksorski L, Rosenberg L. Smell identification ability: Changes with age. *Science.* 1984; 226(4681): 1441–43.

Doty RL. Olfactory dysfunction in Parkinson disease. *Nat Rev Neurol.* 2012; 8(6): 329–39.

Doty RL. The olfactory system and its disorders. *Semin Neurol.* 2009; 29(1): 74–81.

Duff K, McCaffrey RJ, Solomon GS. The pocket smell test: Successfully discriminating probable Alzheimer's dementia from vascular dementia and major depression. *J Neuropsychiatry Clin Neurosci.* 2002; 14(2): 197–201.

Duvernoy HM. *The human brain: Surface, three-dimensional sectional anatomy with MRI and blood supply.* Vienna, Austria: Springer-Verlag; 1999.

Dysken MW, Sano M, Asthana S, et al. Effect of vitamin E and memantine on functional decline in Alzheimer disease: The TEAM-AD VA cooperative randomized trial. *JAMA.* 2014; 311: 33–44. doi:10.1001/jama.2013.282834

Eaton M, Mitchell-Bonair IL, Friedmann E. The effect of touch on nutritional intake of chronic organic brain syndrome patients. *J Gerontol.* 1986 Sep; 41(5): 611–6.

Echenhofer FG, Coombs MM. A brief review of research and controversies in EEG biofeedback and meditation. *J Transpersonal Psychol.* 1987; 19(2): 161–70.

Edelman, G. *The remembered present: A biological theory of consciousness.* New York, NY: Basic Books; 1989.

Eliade M. Recent works on shamanism, A review article. *Hist Religions.* 1961 Summer; 1(1), 152–86.

Elkis H, Buckley PF. Biology of schizophrenia: Is treatment refractoriness synonymous with severity of illness [A.K.A. is this a drug efficacy problem or an expression of severe illness?]. In: Buckley PF, Gaughran F. eds. Treatment-refractory schizophrenia. Berlin, Germany: Springer-Verlag; 2014. doi:10.1007/978-3-642-45257-4_2

Emond V, Joyal C, Poissant H. Structural and functional neuroanatomy of attention-deficit hyperactivity disorder (ADHD). *Encephale.* 2009 April; 35(2): 107–14. doi:10.1016/ j.encep.2008.01.005. Epub 2008 Jul

Escada PA, Lima C, da Silva JM. The human olfactory mucosa. *Eur Arch Otorhinolaryngol.* 2009; 266(11): 1675–80.

Fan J, McCandliss BD, Fossella J, Flombaum JI, Posner MI. The activation of attentional networks. *NeuroImage.*2005 June; 26(2): 471–9.

Farina N, Llewellyn D, Isaac MG, Tabet N. Vitamin E for Alzheimer's dementia and mild cognitive impairment. *Cochrane Database Syst Rev.* 2017; 1: CD002854.

Faucher J, Koszycki D, Bradwejn J, Merali Z, Bielajew C. Effects of CBT versus MBSR treatment on social stress reactions in social anxiety disorder. *Mindfulness.* 2016; 7(2): 514.

Fava GA, Sonino N. The clinical domains of psychosomatic medicine. *J Clin Psychiatry.* 2005 July; 66(7): 849–58.

Feibleman JK. *Aesthetics: A study of the fine arts in theory and practice.* New York, NY: Duell, Sloan and Pearce; 1949.

Fiebach CJ, Schubotz RI. Dynamic anticipatory processing of hierarchical sequential events: A common role for Broca's area and ventral premotor cortex across domains? *Cortex.* 2006; 42: 499–502. [PubMed]

Field T. Yoga clinical research review. *Complement Ther Clin Pract.* 2011 Feb; 17(1): 1–8.

Firuzi O, Praticò D. Coxibs and Alzheimer's disease: Should they stay or should they go? *Ann Neurol.* 2006; 59: 219–28.

Fitzgerald JM, Lawrence R. Autobiographical memory across the lifespan. *J Geron.* 1984; 39: 692–8.

Fitzsimmons L, Shively M, Verderber A. Variables influencing cardiovascular function. *J Cardiovasc Nurs.* 1991; 5(4): 87–9.

Fjorback LO, Arendt M, Ornbøl E, Fink P, Walach H. Mindfulness-based stress reduction and mindfulness-based cognitive therapy: A systematic review of randomized controlled trials. *Acta Psychiatr Scand.* 2011 Aug; 124(2): 102–19.

Fjorback LO, Walach H. Meditation based therapies—A systematic review and some critical observations. *Religions.* 2012; 3(1), 1–18. doi:10.3390/rel3010001

Flavell JH. Metacognition and metacognitive monitoring: A new area of cognitive developmental inquiry. *Am Psychol,* 1979; 34: 906–11.

Fleming A. On the Antibacterial action of cultures of a penicillium, with special reference to their use in the isolation of B. influenzæ. *Br J Exp Pathol.* 1929 June; 10(3): 226–36.

Foster NA, Valentine ER. The effect of auditory stimulation on autobiographical recall in dementia. *Exp Aging Res.* 2001 Jul–Sep; 27(3): 215–28.

Fox MD, Snyder AZ, Vincent JL, Corbetta M, Van Essen DC, Raichle ME. The human brain is intrinsically organized into dynamic, anticorrelated functional networks. *Proc Natl Acad Sci USA.* 2005; 102: 9673–8. [PMC free article] [PubMed]

Fransson P. How default is the default mode of brain function? Further evidence from intrinsic BOLD signal fluctuations. *Neuropsychologia.* 2006; 44: 2836–45.

Freeman WJ. Consciousness, intentionality, and causality. *J. Conscious Stud.* 1999 Nov/Dec; 6: 143–72.

Fromholt P, Mortensen D, Torpdahl P, Bender L, Larsen P, Rubin D. Life narrative and word-cued autobiographical memories in centenarians: Comparisons with 80-year-old control, depressed, and dementia groups. *Memory.* 2003; 11: 81–8.

Galasko D, Hansen LA, Katzman R, et al. Clinical-neuropathological correlations in Alzheimer's disease and related dementias. *Arch Neurol.* 1994; 51: 888–95. doi:10.1001/arch-neur.1994.0054210060013

Galasko DR, Peskind E, Clark CM, et al. Antioxidants for Alzheimer disease: A randomized clinical trial with cerebrospinal fluid biomarker measures. *Arch Neurol.* 2012 July; 69: 836–41. doi:10.1001/archneurol.2012.85

Galvin JE, Powlishta KK, Wilkins K, McKeel DW, Xiong C, Grant E, Storandt M, Morris JC. Predictors of preclinical Alzheimer disease and dementia: A clinicopathologic study. *Arch Neurol.* 2005 May; 62(5): 758–65. doi:10.1001/archneur.62.5.758

Ganguli M, Dodge HH, Shen C, DeKosky ST. Mild cognitive impairment, amnestic type: An epidemiologic study. *Neurology.* 2004 July; 63(1): 115–21.

Gardiner JM. Episodic memory and autonoetic consciousness: A first person approach. *The Royal Society.* 2001; 356: 1351–61.

Gardiner P, Lestoquoy AS, Gergen-Barnett K, Penti B, White LF, Saper R, Fredman L, Stillman S, Negash NL, Adelstein P, Brackup I, Farrell-Riley C, Kabbara K, Laird L, Mitchell S, Bickmore T, Shamekhi A, Liebschutz JM. Design of the integrative medical group visits randomized control trial for underserved patients with chronic pain and depression. *Contemp Clin Trials,* 2017; 54: 25–35.

Gerbarg PL, Wallace G, Brown RP. Mass disasters and mind-body solutions: Evidence and field insights. *Int J Yoga Therap.* 2011; 21: 97–107.

Gethin R. On some definitions of mindfulness. *Contemporary Buddhism: An Interdisciplinary Journal.* 2011; 12(1), 263–79.

Gethin RML. *The Buddhist path to awakening: A study of the Bodhi-Pakkhiyā Dhammā.* Oxford, UK: Oneworld; 2001.

Gierer A. Brain, mind and limitations of a scientific theory of human consciousness. *Bioessays.* 2008 May; 30(5): 499–505.

Gierer A. Brain, mind and limitations of a scientific theory of human consciousness. *Bioessays.* 2008 May; 30(5): 499–505. doi:10.1002/bies.20743

Gilbert SJ, Spengler S, Simons JS, Steele JD, Lawrie SM, Frith CD, Burgess PW. Functional specialization within rostral prefrontal cortex (area 10): A meta-analysis. *J Cogn Neurosci.* 2006; 18: 932–48. [PubMed]

Gilboa A, Winocur G, Grady CL, Hevenor SJ, Moscovitch M. Remembering our past: Functional neuroanatomy of recollection of recent and very remote personal events. *Cereb Cortex.* 2004; 14: 1214–25. [PubMed]

Gilboa A. Autobiographical and episodic memory—one and the same? Evidence from prefrontal activation in neuroimaging studies. *Neuropsychologia.* 2004; 42: 1336–49. [PubMed]

Gilpin R. 2008. The use of Theravāda Buddhist practices and perspectives in mindfulness-based cognitive therapy. *Contemporary Buddhism.* 2008; 9: 227–51.

Glaser R, Sheridan J, Malarkey WB, MacCallum RC, Kiecolt-Glaser JK. (2000). Chronic stress modulates the immune response to a pneumococcal pneumonia vaccine. *Psychosomatic Med,* 2000; 62: 804–7.

Glusker JP. Dorothy Crowfoot Hodgkin (1910–1994). *Protein Sci.* 1994 Dec; 3(12): 2465–9.

Godin G, Shephard RJ. A simple method to assess exercise behavior in the community. *Can J Appl Sport Sci.* 1985; 10: 141–6.

Gogerly D. On Buddhism. *J Ceylon Branch Royal Asiatic Society.* 1845; 1, 7–28.

Gogerly D. The books of discipline. In: Bishop AS. ed. *Ceylon Buddhism being the collected writings of Daniel John Gogerly.* Colombo, Ceylon: Wesleyan Methodist Book Room; 1908: 45–100.

Gokulananda S. *How to overcome mental tension.* West Bengal, India: Ramakrishna Mission Institute of Culture Publisher; 1997.

Gold BT, Buckner RL. Common prefrontal regions coactivate with dissociable posterior regions during controlled semantic and phonological tasks. *Neuron.* 2002; 35: 803–12. [PubMed]

Gold C, Erkkilä J, Crawford MJ. Shifting effects in randomised controlled trials of complex interventions: A new kind of performance bias? *Acta Psychiatr Scand.* 2012; 126(5): 307–14. doi:10.1111/j.1600-0447.2012.01922.x. Epub 2012 Sep 4.

Gordon JL, Rubinow DR, Eisenlohr-Moul TA, Leserman J, Girdler SS. Estradiol variability, stressful life events, and the emergence of depressive symptomatology during the menopausal transition. *Menopause.* 2016; 23(3): 257–66. doi:10.1097/GME. 0000000000000528

Grasset L, Brayne C, Joly P, et al. Trends in dementia incidence: Evolution over a 10-year period in France. *Alzheimers Dement.* 2016 Mar; 12(3): 272–80. doi: 10.1016/j/jalz.2015.11.001. Epub 2015 Dec 13.

Gratz KL, Roemer L. (2004). Multidimensional assessment of emotion regulation and dysregulation: Development, factor structure, and initial validation of the difficulties in emotion regulation scale. *J Psychopath Behav Assess.* 2004; 26(1): 41–54.

Grob HM. Paraverbal psychomotor techniques in neurologic habilitation and rehabilitation. In: Tomaino CM. ed. *Clinical applications of music in neurologic rehabilitation.* St. Louis, MO: MMB Music; 1998: 37–40.

Gross JJ, Carstensen LL, Pasupathi M, Tsai J, Skorpen CG, Hsu AY. Emotion and aging: Experience, expression, and control. *Psychol Aging.* 1997; 12(4): 590–9.

Gross JJ. Emotion regulation: Affective, cognitive, and social consequences. *Psychophysiol.* 2002; 39(3): 281–91.

Gross J-L, Swartz R. The effects of music therapy on anxiety in chronically ill patients. *Music Therapy.* 1982; 2(1): 43–52. doi:10.1093/mt/2.1.43

Grossman P, Niemann L, Schmidt S, Walach H. (2004). Mindfulness-based stress reduction and health benefits: A meta-analysis. *J Psychosomatic Res.* 2004; 57: 35–43.

Grossman P, Van Dam NT. Mindfulness, by any other name…: Trials and tribulations of sati in western psychology and science. *Contemporary Buddhism: An Interdisciplinary Journal.* 2011; 12(1): 219–39.

Guillaumie L, Boiral O, Champagne J. A mixed-methods systematic review of the effects of mindfulness on nurses. *J Adv Nurs.* 2017 May; 73(3): 1017–34. doi:10.1111/jan.13176

Gura ST. Yoga for stress reduction and injury prevention at work. *Work: J Prev, Assess, Rehab.* 2002; 19: 3–7.

Gurjar AA, Ladhake SA, Thakare AP. Analysis of acoustic of "OM" chant to study its effect on nervous system. *Intl J Computer Sci Network Security.* 2009 Jan; 9(1).

Gurjar AA, Ladhake SA. Time frequency analysis of chanting Sanskrit divine sound "OM" mantra. *Intl J Computer Sci Network Security.* 2008 Aug; 8(8): 170–5.

Gusnard DA, Raichle ME. Searching for a baseline: Functional imaging and the resting human brain. *Nat Rev Neurosci.* 2001; 2: 685–94. [PubMed]

Halgren E, Dhond RP, Christensen N, Van Petten C, Marinkovic K, Lewine JD, Dale AM. N400-like magnetoencephalography responses modulated by semantic context, word frequency, and lexical class in sentences. *NeuroImage.* 2002; 17: 1101–16. [PubMed]

Hameroff S, Penrose R. Consciousness in the universe: A review of the 'Orch OR' theory. *Phys Life Rev.* 2014 Mar; 11(1): 39–78.

Handy TC, Miller MB, Schott B, Shroff NM, Janata P, Van Horn JD, Inati S, Grafton ST, Gazzaniga MS. Visual imagery and memory—do retrieval strategies affect what the mind's eye sees? *Eur J Cogn Psychol.* 2004; 16: 631–52.

Haneishi E. Effects of a music therapy voice protocol on speech intelligibility, vocal acoustic measures, and mood of individuals with Parkinson's disease. *J Music Ther.* 2001, Winter; 38(4): 273–90.

Hanney M, Prasher V, Williams N, et al. Memantine for dementia in adults older than 40 years with Down's syndrome (MEADOWS): A randomised, double-blind, placebo-controlled trial. *Lancet.* 2012; 379: 528–36. doi:10.1016/S0140-6736(11)61676-0. Epub 2012 Jan 10.

Harasty JA, Halliday GM, Xuereb J, et al. Cortical degeneration associated with phonologic and semantic language impairments in AD. *Neurology.* 2001 May; 56: 944–50.

Hardy RS. *A manual of Buddhism: In its modern development.* London, UK: Partridge and Oakey; 1853.

Hardy RS. *Eastern monachism.* London, UK: Partridge and Oakey; 1850.

Hare EM, Woodward FL. *The book of the gradual sayings.* 5 vols. London, UK: Pali Text Society; 1932–6.

Harwood DG, Sultzer DL, Feil D, et al. Frontal lobe hypometabolism and impaired insight in Alzheimer disease. *Am J Geriatr Psychiatry.* 2005; 13: 934–41.

Harwood DG, Sultzer DL, Wheatley MV. Impaired insight in Alzheimer disease: Association with cognitive deficits, psychiatric symptoms, and behavioral disturbances. *Neuropsychiatry Neuropsychol Behav Neurol.* 2000; 13(2): 83–88.

Haug HJ, Rössler W. Deinstitutionalization of psychiatric patients in central Europe. *Eur Arch Psychiatry Clin Neurosci.* 1999; 249(3): 115–22.

Hauge CR, Bonde PJE, Rasmussen A, Skovbjerg S. Mindfulness-based cognitive therapy for multiple chemical sensitivity: A study protocol for a randomized controlled trial. *Trials.* 2012; 13, 179. doi:10.1186/1745-6215-13-179

Hauser WA, Morris ML, Heston LL, Anderson VE. Seizures and myoclonus in patients with Alzheimer's disease. *Neurology.* 1986; 36: 1226. doi:10.1212.WNL.36.9.1226

Hawkins HM. *The healing power of music: The Buddha listens to the sound of the universe.* Seattle, WA: Northwest Institute of Acupuncture and Oriental Medicine; 1994.

Haycox JA. A simple, reliable clinical behavioral scale for assessing demented patients. *J Clin Psychiatry.* 1984 Jan; 45(1): 23–4.

Hazlett-Stevens H. Mindfulness-based stress reduction for comorbid anxiety and depression. *J Nerv Ment Dis.* 2012; 200(11): 999–1003. doi:10.1097/NMD.0b013e3182718a61

Herdt J, Bührlen B, Bader K, Hänny C. Participation in an adapted version of MBCT in psychiatric care. *Mindfulness.* 2012; 3(3), 218.

Hertenstein E, Rose N, Voderholzer U, Heidenreich T, Nissen C, Thiel N, Herbst N, Külz AK. Mindfulness-based cognitive therapy in obsessive-compulsive disorder—A qualitative study on patients' experiences. *BMC Psychiatry.* 2012; 12; 185. doi. 10.1186/1471-233X-12-185

Hesslow G. Will neuroscience explain consciousness? *J Theor Biol.* 1994 Nov 7; 171(1): 29–39.

Hillecke T, Nickel A, Bolay HV. Scientific perspectives on music therapy. *Ann N Y Acad Sci.* 2005 Dec; 1060: 271–82.

Hodgins HS, Adair KC. Attentional processes and meditation. *Conscious Cogn.* 2010 Dec; 19(4): 872–8.

Hofmann SG, Sawyer AT, Witt AA, Oh D. Effect of mindfulness-based therapy on anxiety and depression: A meta-analytic review. *J Consult Clin Psychol.* 2010 April; 78(2): 169–83. doi:10.1037/a0018555

Horner IB. *Middle length sayings.* 3 vols. London, UK: Pali Text Society; 1954–9.

Howard R, McShane R, Lindesay J, et al. Donepezil and memantine for moderate-to-severe Alzheimer's disease. *N Engl J Med.* 2012; 366: 893–903.

Howard R, McShane R, Lindesay J, et al. Nursing home placement in the donepezil and memantine in moderate to severe Alzheimer's disease (DOMINO-AD) trial: Secondary and post-hoc analyses. *Lancet Neurol.* 2015; 14: 1171.

Huguelet P, Koenig HG. *Religion and spirituality in psychiatry.* New York, NY: Cambridge University Press; 2017.

Imbimbo BP, Solfrizzi V, Panza F. Are NSAIDs useful to treat Alzheimer's disease or mild cognitive impairment? *Front Aging Neurosci.* 2010; 2: 19. doi:10.3389/fnagi.1020.00019. eCollection 2010

Innes KE, Selfe TK. Meditation as a therapeutic intervention for adults at risk for Alzheimer's disease—potential benefits and underlying mechanisms. *Front Psychiatry.* 2014; 5: 40.

Irizarry MC, Jin S, He F, et al. Incidence of new-onset seizures in mild to moderate Alzheimer disease. *Arch Neurol.* 2012; 69: 368–72. doi:10.1001/archneurol.2011.830

Ivanovski B, Malhi GS. The psychological and neurophysiological concomitants of mindfulness forms of meditation. *Acta Neuropsychiatrica.* 2007; 19(2): 76–91.

Jaffray L, Bridgman H, Stephens M, Skinner T. Evaluating the effects of mindfulness-based interventions for informal palliative caregivers: A systematic literature review. *Palliat Med.* 2016 Feb; 30(2): 117–31. doi:10.1177/0269216315600331. Epub 2015 Aug 17.

Janata P, Birk JL, Tillmann B, Bharucha JJ. Online detection of tonal pop-out in modulating contexts. *Music Percept.* 2003; 20: 283–305.

Janata P, Birk JL, Van Horn JD, Leman M, Tillmann B, Bharucha JJ. The cortical topography of tonal structures underlying Western music. *Science.* 2002; 298: 2167–70.

Janata P, Grafton ST. Swinging in the brain: Shared neural substrates for behaviors related to sequencing and music. *Nat Neurosci.* 2003; 6: 682–7.

Janata P. Brain networks that track musical structure. *Ann N Y Acad Sci.* 2005; 1060: 111–24.

Janata P. Navigating tonal space. In: Hewlett WB, Selfridge-Field E, Correia E. eds. *Tonal theory for the digital age.* Stanford (CA): Center for Computer Assisted Research in the Humanities; 2007–8: 39–50.

Janata P. The neural architecture of music-evoked autobiographical memories. *Cereb Cortex.* 2009 Nov; 19(1): 2579–94.

Jaturapatporn D, Isaac MG, McCleery J, Tabet N. Aspirin, steroidal and non-steroidal anti-inflammatory drugs for the treatment of Alzheimer's disease. *Cochrane Database Syst Rev.* 2012. CD006378.

Jayawardene W, Erbe R, Lohrmann D, Torabi M. Use of treatment and counseling services and mind-body techniques by students with emotional and behavioral difficulties. *J School Health.* 2017; 87(2): 133–41.

Jensen CG, Vangkilde S, Frokjaer V, Hasselbalch SG. Mindfulness training affects attention—or is it attentional effort? *J Exp Psychol Gen.* 2012 Feb; 141(1): 106–23. Epub 2011 Sep 12.

Jevning R, Wallace RK, Beidebach M. The physiology of meditation: A review. A wakeful hypometabolic integrated response. *Neurosci Biobehav Rev.* 1992; 16(3), 415–24.

Jha A, Klein R, Krompinger J, Baime M. Mindfulness training modifies subsystems of attention. *Cogn Affect Behav Neurosci.* 2007 Jun; 7(2): 109–19.

Jones DS. The health care experiments at Many Farms: The Navajo, tuberculosis, and the limits of modern medicine, 1952–1962. *Bull Hist Med.* 2002 Winter; 76(4): 749–90.

Josipovic A. Neural correlates of nondual awareness in meditation. *Ann N Y Acad Sci.* 2014 Jan; 1307: 9–18.

Josipovic Z. Duality and nonduality in meditation research. *Conscious Cog.* 2010; 19(4): 1119–21.

Ju YE, Lucey BP, Holtzman DM. Sleep and Alzheimer disease pathology—a bidirectional relationship. *Nat Rev Neurol.* 2014; 10: 115–9.

Ju YE, McLeland JS, Toedebusch CD, et al. Sleep quality and preclinical Alzheimer disease. *JAMA Neurol* 2013; 70: 587–93. doi:10.1001/jamaneurol.2013.2334

Julian LJ. Measures of anxiety. *Arthritis Care Res* (Hoboken). 2011 Nov; 63 (0 11): 10.1002/acr.20561. doi.10.1002/acr.20561

Kabat-Zinn J, Kabat-Zinn J. Bringing mindfulness to medicine. Interview by Karolyn A. Gazella. *Altern Ther Health Med.* 2005 May–Jun; 11(3): 56–64.

Kabat-Zinn J, Lipworth L, Burney R. The clinical use of mindfulness meditation for the self-regulation of chronic pain. *J Behav Med.* 1985; 8: 163–190.

Kabat-Zinn J, Massion AO, Kristeller J, Peterson LG, Fletcher KE, Pbert L, et al. Effectiveness of a meditation-based stress reduction program in the treatment of anxiety disorders. *Am J Psychiatry.* 1992; 149(7): 936–43.

Kabat-Zinn J, Wheeler E, Light T, Skillings A, Scharf M, Cropley TG, et al. Influence of a mindfulness-based stress reduction intervention on rates of skin clearing in patients with moderate to severe psoriasis undergoing phototherapy (UVB) and photochemotherapy (PUVA). *Psychosomatic Med.* 1998; 60: 625–32.

Kabat-Zinn J. An outpatient program in behavioral medicine for chronic pain based on the practice of mindfulness meditation. *Gen Hosp Psychiatry.* 1982; 4: 33–47.

Kabat-Zinn J. *Full catastrophe living: Using the wisdom of your body and mind to face stress, pain, and illness.* New York, NY: Delacorte Press; 1990.

Kabat-Zinn J. Lipworth L, Burney R. The clinical use of mindfulness meditation for the self-regulation of chronic pain. *J Behav Med.* 1985; 8: 163–90.

Kabat-Zinn J. Mindfulness-based interventions in context: Past, present, and future. *Clin Psychol: Sci Pract.* 2003; 10, 144–56.

Kamei T, Toriumi Y. Kimura H, Ohno S, Kumano H, Kimura K. (2000). Decrease in serum cortisol during yoga exercise is correlated with alpha wave activation. *Percept Mot Skills.* 2000; 90: 1027–32.

Kearns NP, Shawyer F, Brooker JE, Graham AL, Enticott JC, Martin PR, Meadows GN. Does rumination mediate the relationship between mindfulness and depressive relapse? *Psychol Psychother: Theory, Res Pract.* 2016; 89: 1–33.

Kelly BD. Buddhist psychology, psychotherapy and the brain: A critical introduction. *Transcult Psychiatry.* 2008 Mar; 45(1): 5–30.

Khanna S, Greeson JM. A narrative review of yoga and mindfulness as complementary therapies for addiction. *Complement Ther Med.* 2013 Jun; 21(3): 244–52.

Kirtan Kriya: *Practice the 12-minute yoga meditation exercise.* Tucson,AZ: Alzheimer's Research & Prevention Foundation, 20011–17.

Klatt MD, Buckworth J, Malarkey WB. Effects of low-dose mindfulness-based stress reduction (MBSR-ld) on working adults. *Health Educ Behav.* 2009 Jun; 36(3): 601–14.

Knox R. Musical attention training program and alternating attention in brain injury: An initial report. *Music Ther Perspect.* 2003; 21(2); 99–104.

Kok BE, Singer T. Phenomenological fingerprints of four meditations: Differential state changes in affect, mind-wandering, meta-cognition, and interoception before and after daily practice across 9 months of training. *Mindfulness.* 2017; 8(1): 218. Doi:10.1007/s12671-016-0594-9

Kopelman M, Wilson BA, Baddeley A. *The autobiographical memory interview.* Bury St. Edmunds, UK: Thames Valley Test Company; 1990.

Kopelman MD. Rates of forgetting in Alzheimer-type dementia and Korsakoff's syndrome. *Neuropsychologia.* 1985; 15:527–41.

Kornfield J. *Living Buddhist masters.* Santa Cruz, CA: University Press; 1977.

Kornhuber J, Weller M, Schoppmeyer K, Riederer P. Amantadine and memantine are NMDA receptor antagonists with neuroprotective properties. *J Neural Transm Suppl.* 1994; 43: 91–104.

Kozhevnikov M, Louchakova O, Josipovic Z, Motes MA. The enhancement of visuospatial processing efficiency through Buddhist deity meditation. *Psychol Sci.* 2009 May; 20(5): 645–53.

Kuan T-F. *Mindfulness in early Buddhism: New approaches through psychology and textual analysis of Pali, Chinese, and Sanskrit sources.* London, UK: Routledge; 2008.

Kyabgon T. *The benevolent mind: A manual in mind training.* Auckland, NZ: Chyisil Chokyi Gyatsal Trust; 2003.

Lancelot E, Beal MF. Glutamate toxicity in chronic neurodegenerative disease. *Prog Brain Res.* 1998; 116: 331–47.

Lane RD, Quinlan DM, Swartz GE, Walker PA, Zeitlin SB. (1987). The Levels of Emotional Awareness Scale: A cognitive-developmental measure of emotion. J Pers Assess. 1987; 55: 124–34.

Laneri D, Schuster V, Dietsche B, Jansen A, Ott U, Sommer J. Effects of long-term mindfulness meditation on brain's white matter microstructure and its aging. *Front Aging Neurosci.* 2016 Jan 14; 7: 254. https://doi.org/10.3389/fnagi.2015.00254

Lauretti E, Li JG, Di Meco A, Praticò D. Glucose deficit triggers tau pathology and synaptic dysfunction in a tauopathy mouse model. Transl Psychiatry. 2017 Jan 31; 7(1):e1020. doi:10.1038/tp.2016.296

Lazar SW, Kerr CE, Wasserman RH, Gray JR, Greve DN, Treadway MT, McGarvey M, Quinn BT, Dusek JA, Benson H, et al. Meditation experience is associated with increased cortical thickness. *Neuroreport.* 2005 Nov 28; 16(17): 1893–7.

Lee BY. The role of internists during epidemics, outbreaks, and bioterrorist attacks. *J. Gen Intern Med.* 2007 Jan; 22(1): 131–6.

Lee K-H, Lin H-C, Wang P-W, Yen C-F. An integrated model of depression, compulsion, and mindfulness among heroin abusers in Taiwan. *Am J Addict.* 2016; 25(3): 227–32. doi:10.1111/ajad.12365. Epub 2016 Mar 17.

Lestage P, Xu R. Effets de la pratique de la pleine conscience et du Tai Chi Chuan sur la santé mentale d'étudiants: une étude pilote contrôlée non randomisée, *J Thérapie Comportementale Cog*, 2016; 26(1): 32.

Lippelt DP, Hommel B, Colzato LS. Focused attention, open monitoring and loving kindness meditation: Effects on attention, conflict monitoring, and creativity—A review. *Front Psychol.* 2014; 5: 1083. doi:10.3389/fpsyg.2014.01083

Little A. Treatment-resistant depression, *Am Fam Physician.* 2009 Jul 15; 80(2):167–72.

Lockhart RS. Methods of memory research. In Tulving E, Craik FIM. eds. *The Oxford handbook of memory.* Oxford, UK: Oxford University Press; 2000: 45–57.

Loizzo J, Charlson M, Peterson J. A program in contemplative self-healing: Stress, allostasis, and learning in the Indo-Tibetan tradition. *Ann N Y Acad Sci.* 2009 Aug; 1172: 1–24.

Loizzo J. Meditation research, past, present, and future: Perspectives from the Nalanda contemplative science tradition. *Ann N Y Acad Sci.* 2014 Jan; 1307(1): 43–54.

Lombard, DO. Exploring the brain-mind-body connection. Interview by Frank Lampe and Suzanne Snyder. *J Altern Ther Health Med.* 2007 Sep–Oct; 13(5): 66–76.

Lutz A, Brefczynski-Lewis J, Johnstone T, Davidson RJ. Regulation of the neural circuitry of emotion by compassion meditation: Effects of meditative expertise. *PLoS One.* 2008; 3(3): e1897. doi:10.1371/journal.pone.0001897

Lutz A, Brefczynski-Lewis JA, Johnstone T, Davidson RJ. Voluntary regulation of the neural circuitry of emotion by compassion meditation: Effects of expertise. *PLoS One.* 2008; 3(3): e1897.

Lutz A, Dunne JD, Davidson RJ. Meditation and the neuroscience of consciousness. In: Zelazo PD, Moscovitch M, Thompson E. eds. *The Cambridge handbook of consciousness.* Cambridge, UK: Cambridge University Press; 2007: 19–497.

Lutz A, Greischar LL, Rawlings NB, Ricard M, Davidson RJ. (2004). Long-term meditators self-induce high-amplitude gamma synchrony during mental practice. *Proc Natl Acad Sci U S A.* 2004; 101: 16369–73.

Lutz A. Meditation and the neuroscience of consciousness: An introduction. In: Zelazo PD, Moscovitch M, Thompson E. eds. *The Cambridge handbook of consciousness.* New York, NY: Cambridge University Press; 2007: 499–551.

Luu K, Hall PA. Examining the acute effects of hatha yoga and mindfulness meditation on executive function and mood. *Mindfulness.* 2016. doi:10.1007/x12671-016-0661-2

Mah L, Szabuniewicz C, Fiocco AJ. Can anxiety damage the brain? *Curr Opin Psychiatry.* 2016 Jan; 29(1): 56–63.

Mahoney DF, Jones RN, Coon DW, Mendelsohn AB, Gitlin LN, Ory M. The Caregiver Vigilance Scale: Application and validation in the Resources for Enhancing Alzheimer's Caregiver Health (REACH) project. *Am J Alzheimers Dis Other Demen*. 2003 Jan–Feb; 18(1): 39–48.

Marchand WR. Mindfulness-based stress reduction, mindfulness-based cognitive therapy, and Zen meditation for depression, anxiety, pain, and psychological distress. *J Psychiatric Pract*. 2012; 18(4): 233–52. doi:10.1097/01.pra.0000416014.53215.86

Marciniak R, Sherdova K, Čermálová P, Hudeček D, Šumec R, Hort J. Effect of meditation on cognitive functions in context of aging and neurodegenerative diseases. *Front Behav Neurosci*. 2014; 8: 17.

Martin JP. The common factor of mindfulness—An expanding discourse: Comment on Horowitz. *J Psychother Integr*. 2002; 12(2): 139–42.

Mathuyr P. Hand hygiene: Back to the basics of infection control. *Indian J Med Res*. 2011 Nov; 134(5): 611–20.

McAreavey MJ, Ballinger BR, Fenton GW. Epileptic seizures in elderly patients with dementia. *Epilepsia*. 1992; 33: 657–60. doi.10.1111/j.1528-1157.1992.tb02343.x

McCorry LK. Physiology of the autonomic nervous system. *Am J Pharm Ed*. 2007; 71(4), 78.

McDaniel KD, Edland SD, Heyman A. Relationship between level of insight and severity of dementia in Alzheimer disease. CERAD Clinical Investigators. Consortium to Establish a Registry for Alzheimer's Disease. *Alzheimer Dis Assoc Disord*. 1995; 9: 101–4.

McKhann GM, Knopman DS, Chertkow H, et al. The diagnosis of dementia due to Alzheimer's disease: Recommendations from the National Institute on Aging-Alzheimer's Association workgroups on diagnostic guidelines for Alzheimer's disease. *Alzheimers Dement*. 2011; 7: 263.

McShane R, Areosa Sastre A, Minakaran N. Memantine for dementia. *Cochrane Database Syst Rev* 2006; CD003154.

Mega JL, Simon T, Collet J-P, Anderson JL, Antman EM, Bliden K, Cannon CP, Danchin N, Giusti B, Gurbel P, Horne BD, Hulot J-S, Kastrati A, Montalescot G, Neumann F-J, Shen L, Sibbing D, Steg PG, Trenk D, Wiviott SD, Sabatine MD. Reduced-function *CYP2C19* genotype and risk of adverse clinical outcomes among patients treated with clopidogrel predominantly for PCI: A meta-analysis. *JAMA*. 2010 Oct 27; 304(16): 1821–30.

Merdes AR, Hansen LA, Jeste DV, et al. Influence of Alzheimer pathology on clinical diagnostic accuracy in dementia with Lewy bodies. *Neurology*. 2003; 60: 1586–90.

Micozzi MS. *Fundamentals of complementary and integrative medicine*. New York, NY: Saunders Elsevier; 2006.

Millán-Calenti JC, Lorenzo-López L, Alonso-Búa B, de Labra C, González-Abraldes I, Maseda A. Optimal nonpharmacological management of agitation in Alzheimer's disease: Challenges and solutions. *Clin Interv Aging*. 2016; 11: 175–84.

Miller GA. The magical number seven, plus or minus two: Some limits on our capacity for processing information. *Psychol Rev*. 1956; 63: 81–97.

Milner B. Amnesia following operation on the temporal lobes. In Whitty CWM, Zangwill OL. eds. *Amnesia*. London: Butterworth; 1966.

Milton I. What does mindfulness really mean? Therapeutic and liberating effects: Part II. *Psychother Australia*. 2011 Nov; 18(1): 74–8.

Mipham SJ. *1999 Seminary transcripts, Teaching from the Sutra tradition.* Nova Scotia, Canada: Vajradhatu; 2000.

Miyake A, Friedman N, Emerson MJ, Witzki AH, Howerter A, Wager T. The unity and diversity of executive functions and their contributions to complex frontal lobe tasks: A latent variable analysis. *Cogn Psych.* 2000; 41: 49–100.

Mizrahi R, Starkstein SE, Jorge R, Robinson RG. Phenomenology and clinical correlates of delusions in Alzheimer disease. *Am J Geriatr Psychiatry.* 2006; 14: 573–81.

Monier-Williams M. *Sanskrit-English dictionary etymologically and philologically arranged.* Oxford, UK: The Clarendon Press; 1872.

Moore CD, Cohen MX, Ranganath C. Neural mechanisms of expert skills in visual working memory. *J Neurosci.* 2006; 26: 11187–96.

Morse DR, Martin JS, Furst ML, Dubin LL, A physiological and subjective evaluation of meditation, hypnosis, and relaxation. *Psychosom Med.* 1977; 39(5): 304–24.

Morton LL, Kershner JR, Siegel LS. The potential for therapeutic applications of music on problems related to memory and attention. *J Music Ther.* 1990; 27(4): 195–208.

Mueller C, Luehrs M, Baecke S, Adolf D, Luetzkendorf R, Luchtmann M, Nernarding J. Building virtual reality fMRI paradigms: A framework for presenting immersive virtual environments. *J. Neurosci Methods.* 2012 Aug 15; 209(2): 290–8.

Murphy C, Schubert CR, Cruickshanks KJ, Klein BE, Klein R, Nondahl DM. Prevalence of olfactory impairment in older adults. *JAMA.* 2002; 288(18): 2307–12.

Murphy R. The effects of mindfulness meditation vs. progressive relaxation training on stress egocentrism anger and impulsiveness among inmates. *Diss Abstr Intl*: Section B: The Sciences & Engineering. 1995; 55(8): 3596–604.

Nagel T. What is it like to be a bat? *Philosoph Rev.* 1974; 83: 435–50.

Namoli NA. *The path of purification (Visuddhimagga) by Bhadantācariya Buddhaghosa.* Colombo, Ceylon: Semage; 1964.

Naranjano C, Ornstein RE. *On the psychology of meditation.* New York, NY: Viking Press; 1971.

Naranjo JR, Schmidt BMC. Is it me or not me? Modulation of perceptual-motor awareness and visuomotor performance by mindfulness meditation. *Neurosci.* 2012 Jul 30; 13: 88. Epub 2012 Jul 30.

Neilson K, Ftanou M, Monshat K, Salzberg M, Bell S, Kamm MA, Connell W, Knowles SR, Sevar K, Mancuso SG, Castle D. A controlled study of a group mindfulness intervention for individuals living with inflammatory bowel disease. *Inflamm Bowel Dis.* 2016; 22(3). 694–701. doi:10.1097/MIB.0000000000000629

Neisser U. Memory: What are the important questions? In Gruneberg MM, Morris PE, Sykes RN. eds. *Practical aspects of memory.* London, UK: Academic Press; 1978.

Nelson TO, Stuart RB, Howard C, Crowley M. Metacognition and clinical psychology: A preliminary framework for research and practice. *Clin Psychol Psychother.* 1999; 6, 73–79.

Neumann NU, Frasch K. The neurobiological dimension of meditation—results from neuroimagining studies. *Psychother Psychosom Med Psychol.* 2006 Dec; 56(12): 488–92.

Newberg AB, Wintering N, Khalsa DS, Roggenkamp H, Waldman MR. Meditation effects on cognitive function and cerebral blood flow in subjects with memory loss: A preliminary study. *J Alzheimer's Dis.* 2010; 20(2): 517–26.

Newberg AB. The neuroscientific study of spiritual practices. *Front Psychol.* 2014; 5: 215. https://soi.org/10.3389/fpsyg.2014.00215

Ng SY, Villemagne VL, Masters CL, Rowe CC. Evaluating atypical dementia syndromes using positron emission tomography with carbon 11 labeled Pittsburgh Compound B. *Arch Neurol.* 2007; 64: 1140–44. doi.10.1001/archneur.64.8.1140

Nicholls RW. Music and dance guilds in Igede. In: Jackson IV. ed. More than drumming: Essays on African and Afro-Latin American music and musicians. Westport, CT: Greenwood Press; 1985: 93.

Norman DA, Shallice T. Attention to action: willed and automatic control of behaviour. In Davidson RJ, Schwarts GE, Shapiro D. eds. *Consciousness and self-regulation. Advances in Research and Theory.* vol. 4. New York, NY: Plenum; 1986: 1–18.

Nyanaponika. *The heart of Buddhist meditation: A handbook of mental training based on the Buddha's way of mindfulness.* London, UK: Rider & Company; 1962.

Nyanatusita B, Hecker H. *The life of Nyanatiloka Thera.* Kandy, Sri Lanka: Buddhist Publication Society; 2008.

Nyklíček I, Irrmischer M. For whom does mindfulness-based stress reduction work? Moderating effects of personality. *Mindfulness.* 2017. doi:10.1007.x12671-017-0687-0

Oginska-Bulik N. The role of personal and social resources in preventing adverse health outcomes in employees of uniformed professions. *Intl J Occup Med Environ Health,* 2005; 18: 233–40.

Oliveira-Pinto AV, Santos RM, Coutinho RA, et al. Sexual dimorphism in the human olfactory bulb: females have more neurons and glial cells than males. *PLoS One.* 2014; 9(11): e111733.

Orrego F, Villanueva S. The chemical nature of the main central excitatory transmitter: a critical appraisal based upon release studies and synaptic vesicle localization. *Neurosci.* 1993; 56: 539–55.

Pardini M, Huey ED, Cavanagh AL, Grafman J. Olfactory function in corticobasal syndrome and frontotemporal dementia. *Arch Neurol.* 2009; 66(1): 92–6.

Pelled E. Learning from experience: Bion's concept of reverie and Buddhist meditation. A comparative study. *Int J Psychoanal.* 2007 Dec; 88(Pt 6): 1507–26.

Petersen RC, Smith GE, Waring SC, et al. Mild cognitive impairment: Clinical characterization and outcome. *Arch Neurol.* 1999; 56: 303–8.

Petersen RC, Stevens JC, Ganguli M, et al. Practice parameter: Early detection of dementia—mild cognitive impairment (an evidence-based review). Report of the Quality Standards Subcommittee of the American Academy of Neurology. *Neurology* 2001; 56: 1133–42.

Petersen RC. Clinical practice. Mild cognitive impairment. *N Engl J Med.* 2011; 364: 2227–34. doi.10.1056/NEJMcp0910237

Petersen RC. Conceptual overview. In: Petersen RC. ed. *Mild cognitive impairment: Aging to Alzheimer's disease.* New York, NY: Oxford University Press; 2003.

Petersen RC. Mild cognitive impairment as a diagnostic entity. *J Intern Med.* 2004; 256: 183–94.

Petersen RC. Mild cognitive impairment. *Continuum: Lifelong Learning in Neurology.* 2016 April; 22(2): 40418. doi.10.1212/CON.0000000000000313

Petersen SE, Posner MI. The attention system of the human brain: 20 years after. *Ann Rev Neurosci.* 2012; 35: 73–89.

Pizzagalli DA. Psychobiology of the intersection and divergence of depression and anxiety. *Depress Anxiety.* 2016 Oct; 33(10): 891–94.

Plailly J, Tillmann B, Royet J-P. The feeling of familiarity of music and odors: The same neural signature? *Cereb Cortex.* 2007; 17: 2650–58.

Platel H, Baron JC, Desgranges B, Bernard F, Eustache F. Semantic and episodic memory of music are subserved by distinct neural networks. *NeuroImage.* 2003; 20: 244–56.

Poldrack RA. Neural systems for perceptual skill learning. *Behav Cognit Neurosci Rev.* 2002; 1(1): 76–83.

Porsteinsson AP, Grossberg GT, Mintzer J, et al. Memantine treatment in patients with mild to moderate Alzheimer's disease already receiving a cholinesterase inhibitor: A randomized, double-blind, placebo-controlled trial. *Curr Alzheimer Res* 2008; 5: 83–9.

Posner MI. Orienting of attention. *Q J Exp Psychol.* 1980; 32(1): 3–25.

Potter LT. Discovery of treatments for Alzheimer's disease. *Neurobiol Aging,* 1994; 15 Suppl 2: S67.

Prinsley D. Music therapy in geriatric care. *Aust Nurses J.* 1986; 15(9), 48–9.

Qaseem A, Snow V, Cross JT, et al. Current pharmacologic treatment of dementia: A clinical practice guideline from the American College of Physicians and the American Academy of Family Physicians. *Ann Intern Med.* 2008; 148: 370.

Rahayel S, Frasnelli J, Joubert S. The effect of Alzheimer's disease and Parkinson's disease on olfaction: A meta-analysis. *Behav Brain Res.* 2012; 231: 60–74. doi:10.1016/j.bbr. 2012.03.047. Epub 2012 Mar 5.

Rahe RH, Taylor CB, Tolles RL, Newhall LM, Veach TL, Bryson S. A novel stress and coping workplace program reduces illness and healthcare utilization. *Psychosom Med.* 2002; 64: 278–86.

Raina P, Santaguida P, Ismaila A, et al. Effectiveness of cholinesterase inhibitors and memantine for treating dementia: Evidence review for a clinical practice guideline. *Ann Intern Med.* 2008; 148: 379–97.

Raub JA. Psychophysiologic effects of hatha yoga on musculoskeletal and cardiopulmonary function: A literature review. National Center for Environmental Assessment, Rep. No. 8. Research Triangle Park, NC: National Center for Environmental Assessment; 2002.

Reibel DK, Greeson JM, Brainard GC, Rosenzweig S. Mindfulness-based stress reduction and health-related quality of life in a heterogeneous patient population. *Gen Hosp Psychiatry.* 2001; 23: 183–92.

Reidbord SP. A brief history of psychiatry. Retrieved from http://www.stevenreidbordmd.com/history-of-psychiatry/

Reines SA, Block GA, Morris JC, et al. Rofecoxib: No effect on Alzheimer's disease in a 1-year, randomized, blinded, controlled study. *Neurology.* 2004; 62: 66–71.

Reisberg B, Doody R, Stöffler A, et al. A 24-week open-label extension study of memantine in moderate to severe Alzheimer disease. *Arch Neurol.* 2006; 63: 49–54.

Reisberg B, Doody R, Stöffler A, et al. Memantine in moderate-to-severe Alzheimer's disease. *N Engl J Med.* 2003; 348: 1333–41.

Remington R. Calming music and hand massage with agitated elderly. *Nurs Res.* 2002 Sep–Oct; 51(5): 317–23.

Rhys Davids CAF, Woodward FL. *The book of the kindred sayings*. 5 vols. London, UK: Pali Text Society; 1917–30.

Rhys Davids TW. *Buddhist suttas*. Oxford, UK: Clarendon Press; 1881

Ridgway GR, Lehmann M, Barnes J, et al. Early-onset Alzheimer disease clinical variants: Multivariate analyses of cortical thickness. *Neurology*. 2012; 79:80–84. doi:10.1212/ WNL.0b013e31825dce28

Ritchie K, Artero S, Touchon J. Classification criteria for mild cognitive impairment: A population-based validation study. *Neurology*. 2001; 56: 37–42. doi.10.1212/WNL.56.1.37

Roberts AC, Robbins TW, Weiskrantz L. *The prefrontal cortex: Executive and cognitive functions*. Oxford, UK: Oxford University Press; 1998.

Robins Wahlin TB, Byrne GJ. Personality changes in Alzheimer's disease: A systematic review, *Int J Geriatr Psychiatry*. 2011 Oct; 26(10): 1019–29.

Rogers J, Kirby LC, Hempelman SR, et al. Clinical trial of indomethacin in Alzheimer's disease. Neurology 1993; 43: 1609–11.

Romanelli MF, Morris JC, Ashkin K, Coben LA. Advanced Alzheimer's disease is a risk factor for late-onset seizures. *Arch Neurol*. 1990; 47: 847–50.

Rubin DC. *Memory in oral traditions: The cognitive psychology of epic ballads and counting-out rhymes*. New York, NY: Oxford University Press; 1995.

Ryan L, Nadel L, Keil K, Putnam K, Schnyer D, Trouard T, Moscovitch M. Hippocampal complex and retrieval of recent and very remote autobiographical memories: Evidence from functional magnetic resonance imaging in neurologically intact people. *Hippocampus*. 2001; 11: 707–14.

Ryman DC, Acosta-Baena N, Aisen PS, et al. Symptom onset in autosomal dominant Alzheimer disease: A systematic review and meta-analysis. *Neurology* 2014; 83: 253–60. doi.10.1212/WNL .0000000000000596

Sabatine MS, Cannon CP, Gibson CM, López-Sendón JL, Montalescot G, Theroux P, Lewis BS, Murphy SA, McCabe CH, Braunwald E. Clopidogrel as Adjunctive Reperfusion Therapy (CLARITY)-Thrombolysis in Myocardial Infarction (TIMI) 28 investigator effect of clopidogrel pretreatment before percutaneous coronary intervention in patients with ST-elevation myocardial infarction treated with fibrinolytics: The PCI-CLARITY study. *JAMA*. 2005 Sep 14; 294(10): 1224–32.

Safire W. On language: Proof pudding. *NYT,* 2008 Oct 19.

Salmon D, Hodges JR. Introduction: Mild cognitive impairment—cognitive, behavioral, and biological factors. *Neurocase*. 2005; 11: 1–2.

Sano M, Ernesto C, Thomas RG, et al. A controlled trial of selegiline, alpha-tocopherol, or both as treatment for Alzheimer's disease: The Alzheimer's Disease Cooperative Study. *N Engl J Med*. 1997; 336: 1216–22.

Sano M, Ernesto C, Thomas RG, Klauber MR, Schafer K, Grundman M, Woodbury P, Growdon J, Cotman CW, Pfeiffer E, Schneider LS, Thal LJ. A controlled trial of selegiline, alpha-tocopherol, or both as treatment for Alzheimer's disease. The Alzheimer's Disease Cooperative Study. *N Engl J Med*. 1997 Apr 24; 336(17): 1216–22.

Satizabal CL, Beiser AS, Chouraki V, et al. Incidence of dementia over three decades in the Framingham Heart Study. *N Engl J Med*. 2016; 374: 523–32.

Savona-Ventura C. Hospitaller activities in Medieval Malta. *Malta Med J*. 2007; 19: 48–52.

Scarmeas N, Honig LS, Choi H, et al. Seizures in Alzheimer disease: Who, when, and how common? *Arch Neurol.* 2009; 66: 992–97. doi:10.1001/archneurol.2009.130

Schacter DL. Priming and multiple memory systems: Perceptual mechanisms of implicit memory. In Schacter DL, Tulving E. eds. *Memory systems.* Cambridge, MA: MIT Press; 1994.

Scharf S, Mander A, Ugoni A, et al. A double-blind, placebo-controlled trial of diclofenac/ misoprostol in Alzheimer's disease. *Neurology.* 1999; 53: 197–201.

Schmidt SJ. Mindfulness and healing intention: concepts, practice, and research evaluation. *Altern Complement Med.* 2004; 10 Suppl 1: S7–14.

Schmitz TW, Johnson SC. Relevance to self: A brief review and framework of neural systems underlying appraisal. *Neurosci Biobehav Rev.* 2007; 31: 585–96.

Schneider LS, Dagerman KS, Higgins JP, McShane R. Lack of evidence for the efficacy of memantine in mild Alzheimer disease. *Arch Neurol.* 2011; 68: 991–98. doi:10.1001/archneurol.2011.69

Schulz R, Burgio L, Burns R, Eisdorfer C, Gallagher-Thompson D, Gitlin LN, Mahoney DF. Resources for Enhancing Alzheimer's Caregiver Health (REACH): Overview, site-specific outcomes, and future directions. *Gerontologist.* 2003 Aug; 43(4): 514–20.

Schulz R, McGinnis KA, Zhang S, Martire LM, Hebert RS, Beach SR, Zdaniuk B, Czaja SJ, Belle SH. Dementia patient suffering and caregiver depression. *Alzheimer Dis Assoc Disord.* 2008 April–June; 22(2): 170–6.

Schupf N, Kapell D, Nightingale B, et al. Earlier onset of Alzheimer's disease in men with Down syndrome. *Neurology.* 1998; 50: 991–5.

Scott KM. Prevention of CVD in depression. In: Baune BT, Tully PJ. eds. *Cardiovascular diseases and depression: Treatment and prevention in psychocardiology.* Cham, Switzerland: Springer: 2016; 509–18.

Searle JR. How to study consciousness scientifically. *Philos Trans R Soc Lond B Biol Sci.* 1998 Nov 29; 353(1377): 1935–42.

Searle JR. Minds, brains and programs. *Behav Brain Sci.* 1980; 3: 417–57.

Searle JR. *Minds, brains and science.* Cambridge, MA: Harvard University Press; 1984.

Searle JR. *The rediscovery of the mind.* Cambridge, MA: MIT Press; 1992.

Serby M, Larson P, Kalkstein D. The nature and course of olfactory deficits in Alzheimer's disease. *Am J Psychiatry.* 1991; 148(3): 357–60.

Shah B, Pattanayak RD; Sagar R. The study of patient Henry Molaison and what it taught us over past 50 years: Contributions to neuroscience. *J Mental Health Hum Behav* [serial online]. 2014 [cited 2017 May 10]; 19: 91–3.

Shallice T, Burgess P. (1996). The domain of supervisory processes and temporal organization of behaviour. *Philos Trans R Soc Lond B Biol Sci.* 1996; 351(1346): 1405–11.

Shallice T, Warrington EK. Independent functioning of verbal memory stores: a neuropsychological study. *Q J Exp Psychol.* 1970; 22: 261–73.

Shallice, T. *From neuropsychology to mental structure.* Cambridge, UK: Cambridge University Press; 1988.

Shapiro SL, Oman D, Thoresen CE, Plante TG, Flinders T. Cultivating mindfulness: Effects on well-being. *J Clin Psychol.* 2008 July; 64(7): 840–62.

Shapiro SL, Schwartz GE. The role of intention in self-regulation: Toward intentional systemic mindfulness. In Boekaerts M, Pintrich P. eds. *Handbook of self-regulation*. San Diego, CA: Academic Press; 2000: 253–73.

Sharma VK, Trakroo M, Subramaniam V, Rajajeyakumar M, Bhavanani SB, Sahai A. Effect of fast and slow pranayama on perceived stress and cardiovascular parameters in young health-care students, *Int J Yoga*. 2013 July–Dec; 6(2): 104–10.

Shear J, Mukherjee SP. *Consciousness: A deeper scientific search*. West Bengal, India: Ramakrishna Mission Institute of Culture Publisher; 2006.

Shear J, Mukherjee SP. *Consciousness: A deeper scientific search*. West Bengal, India: Vendata Press of Ramakrishna Institute of Culture; 2007.

Shibles W. Metaphor, music and humor. In: Lehrer K. ed. *Emotion in aesthetics*. Norwell, MA: Kluwer Academic Publishers; 1995: 146–71.

Siegler IC, Welsh KA, Dawson DV, Fillenbaum GG, Earl NL, Kaplan EB, Clark CM. Ratings of personality change in patients being evaluated for memory disorders. *Alzheimer Dis Assoc Disord*. 1991 Winter; 5(4): 240–50.

Silananda U. *The four foundations of mindfulness*. Boston, MA: Wisdom Publications, 1990.

Skovbjerg S, Hauge CR, Rasmussen A, Winkel P, Elberling J. Mindfulness-based cognitive therapy to treat multiple chemical sensitivities: A randomized pilot trial. *Scand J Psychol*. 2012; 53(3): 233–8. doi:10.1111/j.1467-9450.2012.00950.x. Epub.2012 Apr 25.

Slagter HA, Lutz A, Greischar LL, Francis AD, Nieuwenhuis S, Davis JM, Davidson RJ. Mental training affects distribution of limited brain resources. *PLoS Biol*. 2007; 5(6): e138.

Smith BB. *Reclaiming dignity and enhancing abilities through therapeutic stimulation*. Project briefs. Logan, UT: Sunshine Terrace Adult Day Care Center; 1995.

Smith JA, Greer T, Sheets T, Watson S, Stella F, Radanovic M, Balthazar M. Is there more to yoga than exercise? *Altern Ther Health Med*. 2011 May–Jun; 17(3): 22–9.

Snowden J. Disorders of semantic memory. In: Baddeley Ad, Kopelman MD, Wilson BA. eds. *The handbook of memory disorders,* 2nd ed. Chichester, UK: Wiley; 2002: 293–314.

Spira AP, Gamaldo AA, An Y, et al. Self-reported sleep and β-amyloid deposition in community-dwelling older adults. *JAMA Neurol*. 2013; 70(12): 1537–43. doi:10.1001/jamaneurol.2013.4258

Squire LR. The legacy of patient H.M. for neuroscience. *Neuron*. 2009 Jan 15; 61(1): 6–9.

Stamps JJ, Bartoshuk LM, Heilman KM. A brief olfactory test for Alzheimer's disease. *J Neurol Sci*. 2013; 333(1–2): 19–24. doi:10.1016/j.jns.2013.06.033. Epub 2013 Aug 5.

Stanford EP. *Best practice in music therapy: Utilizing group percussion strategies for promoting volunteerism in the well older adult*. (final report) San Diego, CA: University Center on Aging, San Diego State University Foundation; 1995.

Stigsby B, Rodenburg JC, Moth HB. Electroencephalographic findings during mantra meditation (Transcendental Meditation): A controlled, quantitative study of experienced meditators. *Electroencephalogr Clin Neurophysiol*. 1981 April; 51(4): 434–42.

Sun GH, Raji CA, Maceachern MP, Burke JF. Olfactory identification testing as a predictor of the development of Alzheimer's dementia: A systematic review. *Laryngoscope*. 2012; 122: 1455–62. doi:10.1002/lary.23365. Epub 2012 May 2.

Svoboda E, McKinnon MC, Levine B. The functional neuroanatomy of autobiographical memory: A meta-analysis. *Neuropsychologia.* 2006; 44: 2189–2208.

Tang Y, Ma Y, Wang J, Fan Y, Feng S, Lu Q, Yu Q, Sui D, Rothbart MK, Fan M, Posner MI. Short-term meditation training improves attention and self-regulation. *Proc Natl Acad Sci U S A.* 2007 Oct 23; 104(43): 17152–56.

Tariot PN, Farlow MR, Grossberg GT, et al. Memantine treatment in patients with moderate to severe Alzheimer disease already receiving donepezil: A randomized controlled trial. *JAMA.* 2004; 291: 317–24. doi:10.1001/jama.291.3.317

Taylor GJ. Mind-body-environment: George Engel's psychoanalytic approach to psychosomatic medicine. *Aust N Z J Psychiatry.* 2002 Aug; 36(4): 449–57.

Teasdale JD. (1999). Metacognition, mindfulness and the modification of mood disorders. *Clin Psychol Psychother.* 1999; 6: 146–55.

Tennant C. Work-related stress and depressive disorders. *J Psychosom Res,* 2001; 51: 697–704.

Thera N. *The heart of Buddhist meditation: A handbook of mental training based on the Buddha's way of mindfulness.* London, UK: Rider and Company; 1962.

Thiel CM, Zilles K, Fink GR. Cerebral correlates of alerting, orienting and reorienting of visuospatial attention: An event-related fMRI study. *Neuroimage.* 2004 Jan; 21(1): 318–28.

Thompson PM, Hayashi KM, de Zubicaray G, Janke AL, Rose SE, Semple J, Herman D, Hong MS, Dittmer SS, Doddrell DM, et al. Dynamics of gray matter loss in Alzheimer's disease. *J Neurosci.* 2003; 23: 994–1005.

Tillmann B, Janata P, Bharucha JJ. Activation of the inferior frontal cortex in musical priming. *Cognit Brain Res.* 2003; 16: 145–61.

Toiviainen P, Alluri V, Brattico E, Wallentin M, Vuust P. Capturing the musical brain with Lasso: Dynamic decoding of musical features from fMRI data. Neuroimage. 2014 Mar; 88: 170–80.

Toiviainen P, Krumhansl CL. Measuring and modeling real-time responses to music: The dynamics of tonality induction. *Perception.* 2003; 32: 741–66.

Tomic ST, Janata P. Ensemble: A web-based system for psychology survey and experiment management. *Behav Res Methods.* 2007; 39: 635–50.

Trousselard M, Steiler D, Claverie D, Canini F. The history of mindfulness put to the test of current scientific data: Unresolved questions. *Encephale.* 2014 Dec; 40(6): 474–80. Epub 2014 Sep 5.

Tudor M, Tudor L, Tudor KI. Odjel za neurokirurgiju, Klinicka bolnica Split, Split, Hrvatska. [Hans Berger (1873–1941)—the history of electroencephalography]. *Acta Med Croatica.* 2005; 59(4): 307–13.

Tulving E, Craik FIM. *Handbook of memory.* Oxford, UK: Oxford University Press; 2000.

Tulving E, Patkau JE. Concurrent effects of contextual constraint and word frequency on immediate recall and learning of verbal material. *Can J Psychol.* 1962; 16: 83–95.

Vallar G, Baddeley AD. Fractionation of working memory: Neuropsychological evidence for a phonological short-term store. *J Verbal Learning Verbal Behav.* 1984; 23: 151–61.

Vallar G, Papagno C. Neuropsychological impairments of verbal short-term memory. In Baddeley AD, Kopelman MD, Wilson BA. eds. *The handbook of memory disorders.* 2nd ed. Chichester, UK: Wiley; 2002: 249–70.

van der Flier WM, Pijnenburg YA, Fox NC, Scheltens P. Early-onset versus late-onset Alzheimer's disease: The case of the missing APOE ε4 allele. *Lancet Neurol.* 2011; 10(3): 280–88. doi:10.1016/S1474-4422(10)70306-9

van der Klink JJ, Blonk RW, Schene AH, van Dijk FJ. The benefits of interventions for work-related stress. *Am J Public Health.* 2001: 91: 270–76.

Van Gool WA, Weinstein HC, Scheltens P, Walstra GJ. Effect of hydroxychloroquine on progression of dementia in early Alzheimer's disease: An 18-month randomised, double-blind, placebo-controlled study. Lancet. 2001; 358: 455–60. doi:10.1016/S0140-6736(01)05623.9

van Vugt MK, van den Hurk PM. Modeling the effects of attentional cueing on meditators. *Mindfulness.* 2017; 8(1): 38–45. Epub 2016 Jan 9

Vargha-Khadem F, Gadian D, Mishkin M. Dissociations in cognitive memory: The syndrome of developmental amnesia. In Baddeley A, Conway M, Aggleton J. eds. *Episodic memory.* Oxford, UK: Oxford University Press; 2002: 153–63.

Velayudhan L. Smell identification function and Alzheimer's disease: A selective review. *Curr Opin Psychiatry.* 2015; 28(2): 173–79.

Vink AC, Birks JS, Bruinsma MS, Scholten RJ. Music therapy for people with dementia. *Cochrane Database Syst Rev.* 2004; 3: CD003477.

Vink AC, Bruinsma MS, Scholten RJPM. Music therapy for people with dementia. *Cochrane Database Syst Rev.* 2004; (3): CD003477.

Vivek KS, Rajajeyakumar M, Velkumary S, Subramanian SK, Bhacanani AB, Madanmohan AS, Thangavel D. Effect of fast and slow pranayama practice on cognitive functions in healthy volunteers. *J Clin Diagn Res.* 2014 Jan; 8(1): 10–13.

Voisin T, Touchon J, Vellas B. Mild cognitive impairment: A nosological entity? *Curr Opin Neurol.* 2003; 16 Suppl 2: S43-S45.

Wagner AD, Pare-Blagoev EJ, Clark J, Poldrack RA. Recovering meaning: Left prefrontal cortex guides controlled semantic retrieval. *Neuron.* 2001; 31: 329-38.

Walton KG, Schneider RH, Nidich S. Review of controlled research on the transcendental meditation program and cardiovascular disease: Risk factors, morbidity, and mortality. *Cardiol Rev.* 2004 Sep–Oct; 12(5): 262–6.

Warrington EK, Weiskrantz L. New methods of testing long-term retention with special reference to amnesic patients. *Nature.* 1968; 217: 972–974.

Wechsler D. *Wechsler Memory Scale—Revised.* San Antonio, TX: The Psychological Corporation; 1987.

Weiner MF, Hynan LS, Parikh B, et al. Can Alzheimer's disease and dementias with Lewy bodies be distinguished clinically? *J Geriatr Psychiatry Neurol.* 2003 Dec; 16(4): 245-50.

Wells RE, Kerr CE, Wolki J, Dossett M, Davis RB, Walsh J, Wall R, Kong J, Kaptchuk T, Press D, Phillips RS, Yeh G. Meditation for adults with mild cognitive impairment: A pilot randomized trial. *J Am Geriatr Soc.* 2013 Apr; 61(4): 642-5.

West J, Otte C, Geher K, Johnson J, Mohr DC. Effects of hatha yoga and African dance on perceived stress, affect, and salivary cortisol. *Ann Behav Med.* 2004; 28: 114–18.

Westlye LT, Grydeland H, Walhovd KB, Fjell AM. Associations between regional cortical thickness and attentional networks as measured by the attention network test. *Cereb Cortex.* 2011 Feb; 21(2): 345–56.

Wheeler B. *Music therapy research: Quantitative and qualitative perspectives.* New Braunfels, TX: Barcelona Publishers; 1995.

Wheeler BL. Effects of number of sessions and group or individual music therapy on the mood and behavior of people who have had strokes or traumatic brain injuries. *Nordic J Music Ther.* 2003; 12(2): 139–51.

White H, Pieper C, Schmader K, Fillenbaum G. Weight change in Alzheimer's disease. *J Am Geriatr Soc.* 1996 Mar; 44(3): 265–72.

Whitwell JL, Dickson DW, Murray ME, et al. Neuroimaging correlates of pathologically defined subtypes of Alzheimer's disease: A case-control study. *Lancet Neurol.* 2012; 11(10): 868–77. doi:10.1016/S1474-4422(12)70200-4

Wigram AL. Music therapy: Developments in mental handicap. Special Issue: Music therapy. *Psychol Music.* 1988; 16(1): 42–51.

Wigram T, Saperston B, West R. *Art and science of music therapy.* Reading, UK: Harwood Academic Publishers; 1995a.

Wigram T, Saperston B, West R. *The art and science of music therapy: A handbook.* Reading, UK: Harwood Academic Publishers; 1995b.

Wiist WH, Sullivan BM, Wayment HA, Warren M. A web-based survey of the relationship between Buddhist religious practices, health, and psychological characteristics: Research methods and preliminary results. *J Relig Health.* 2010 Mar; 49(1): 18–31.

Wilson B, Cockburn J, Baddeley A, Hiorns R. (1989). The development and validation of a test battery for detecting and monitoring everyday memory problems. *J Clin Exp Neuropsychol,* 1989; 11: 855–70.

Wilson BA, Alderman N, Burgess P, et al. *Behavioural assessment of the dysexecutive syndrome.* Bury St Edmunds, UK: Thames Valley Test Company; 1996.

Wilson BA. Long-term prognosis of patients with severe memory disorders. *Neuropsychol Rehab.* 1991; 1: 117–34.

Wilson RS, Arnold SE, Schneider JA, Tang Y, Bennett DA. The relationship between cerebral Alzheimer's disease pathology and odour identification in old age. *J. Neurol Neurosurg Psychiatry.* 2007; 78: 30–35. doi:10.1136/jnnp.2006.099721.